G000122691

Oral Disease

Oral Disease

edited by

C. E. RENSON

PH.D, BDS, DDPH, LDSRCS

Professor of Conservative Dentistry,
University of Hong Kong.

Formerly Reader in Conservative Dentistry, The
London Hospital Medical College Dental School,
University of London.

1978
UPDATE BOOKS

Published by

UPDATE PUBLICATIONS LTD

Available in the United Kingdom and Eire from

Update Publications Ltd
33/34 Alfred Place
London WC1E 7DP
England

Available outside the United Kingdom from

Update Publishing International, Inc.
2337 Lemoine Avenue
Fort Lee, New Jersey 07024
U.S.A.

First published 1978

British Library Cataloguing in Publication Data

Oral disease.
1. Mouth — Diseases
I. Renson, C E
616.3'1   RC815
ISBN 0-906141-04-4

© Update Publications Ltd, 1978

All rights reserved. No part of this publication may
be reproduced, stored in a retrieval system, or
transmitted, in any form or by any means, elec-
tronic, mechanical, photocopying, recording or
otherwise without the prior permission of the copy-
right owner.

ISBN 0 906141 04 4

Typeset in Great Britain by George Over Ltd,
London and Rugby

Printed in Great Britain by William Clowes & Sons Limited
London, Beccles and Colchester

Contents

Diseases of the Oral Mucosa and Jaws

Neoplasms in the Mouth

Looking at the Throat

List of Contributors

D. S. Berman, PH.D, M.SC, BDS, D.ORTH, DDPH, LDSRCS
Professor of Child Dental Health, The London
Hospital Medical College Dental School, University
of London.

J. Lozdan, BDS, FDSRCS
Formerly Lecturer in Oral Medicine, The London
Hospital Medical College Dental School, University
of London.

D. A. McGowan, MDS, FDSRCS, FFDRCS
Professor of Oral Surgery, Department of Oral and
Maxillo-Facial Surgery, The Dental School,
University of Glasgow.

R. F. McNab Jones, MB, BS, FRCS
Consultant Surgeon in the Ear, Nose and Throat
Department, St. Bartholomew's Hospital, and Royal
National Throat, Nose and Ear Hospital, London.

C. C. Rachanis, BA, B.SC, MB, CH.B, BDS, FDSRCPS
Formerly Lecturer in Oral Medicine, The London
Hospital Medical College Dental School, now at the
University of Witwatersrand Oral and Dental
Hospital, Johannesburg, South Africa.

C. E. Renson, PH.D, BDS, DDPH, LDSRCS
Formerly Reader in Conservative Dentistry, The
London Hospital Medical College Dental School,
University of London, now Professor of Conservative
Dentistry, University of Hong Kong.

G. R. Seward, MB, BS, MDS, FDSRCS
Professor of Oral Surgery, Department of Oral and
Maxillo-Facial Surgery, The London Hospital
Medical College Dental School, University of
London.

D. Stenhouse, MDS, FDSRCS
Senior Lecturer in Dental Surgery, University of
Glasgow.

P. Vig, PH.D, BDS, FDS, D.ORTH, RCS, FRACDS
Formerly Reader in Orthodontics, The London
Hospital Medical College Dental School, University
of London, now Professor of Orthodontics, The
Dental School, University of North Carolina, Chapel
Hill, USA.

Preface

This book is based largely upon a series of articles which originally appeared in *Update*. The purpose of the series was to give medical practitioners an insight into dental and oral disease. The diagnosis of oral disease is not a subject which receives particular emphasis in most medical curricula and it is almost completely absent from many. Postgraduate courses in this field are not generally available to medical practitioners. The prevention and early detection of dental and oral disease can be a very positive contribution to the health of our patients. The dental profession sees only about half the population on a regular basis, though it has been shown that over 99 per cent of the population will suffer from oral disease at some time. This places the burden of responsibility on the shoulders of the medical practitioner.

There are many diseases which originate in and are peculiar to the oral cavity. Many systemic diseases have their early visible manifestations in this area. The early detection and identification of disease and deformity of the oral cavity is an important part of diagnosis in the field of general medicine.

The book is designed to present basic knowledge about the diseases found in the mouth, which will aid in their early recognition, prompt referral and treatment. It is intended as a contribution to disease prevention by taking advantage of the opportunities that fall to medical graduates and undergraduates to draw the attention of patients to conditions that could benefit from medical or dental care.

Dental disease is largely preventable. Tooth loss due to dental caries and gum disease is not inevitable; with proper care there is no reason why patients should not retain a healthy dentition throughout life. In recent years dentistry has made great strides in the prevention and treatment of oral disease. Many disfiguring conditions which were virtually untreatable only a few years ago can now be treated with great success.

The book will also provide the dental student and the operating dental ancilliary with a basis for clinical work and for further reading. It should provide the dental practitioner with a useful revision text and supply him with pictorial reminders of conditions which he may not have seen for some time, perhaps since his student days at dental school. Here the profuse colour illustrations, a special feature of the book, should prove to be particularly helpful. The general principles of management of conditions are suggested but detailed methods of treatment are not included.

Most of the authors of the original series were members of The London Hospital Medical College Dental School, but, with two exceptions, they are now scattered far and wide.

I take this opportunity to acknowledge our debt to the Venereology Department of The London Hospital for their help with some of the illustrations.

A special word of thanks is due to two of my former students, Miss Janice Fiske and Mr Michael Goorwitch for producing the excellent index.

I am indebted to the staff of Update Publications, particularly Dr William Jackson, Mr John Snow, Mr Alan Savill and Miss Christine Drummond for their help with this book.

C. E. Renson

Section 1
Developmental Defects of the Mouth and Jaws

1. The Teeth

David S. Berman

Many developmental anomalies or defects of the primary and permanent dentitions become evident in childhood. The general practitioner may be the first person consulted by the parent. Recognition of an anomaly and subsequent referral of the child for advice can often save anxiety on the part of the parent. In the case of disfiguring conditions referral may avoid an emotionally traumatic situation for the child.

Anomalies can occur in the timing and positioning of the teeth besides defects in their number and structure and colour. Often several defects may occur in one dentition.

Timing and Positioning
Deciduous Dentition

The deciduous or primary dentition is made up of 20 teeth—10 in each arch. The teeth of each arch, incisors, canines and first and second primary molars, may be spaced or in contact (Figure 1.1). The approximate dates of tooth eruption are given in Figure 1.2.

The first teeth to erupt are the lower central incisors at the age of six months. Occasionally a lower central incisor will be present in the mouth at birth and is called a neonatal tooth. Teeth that erupt within a few weeks of birth are termed natal teeth. Such teeth are not fully calcified, they

may or may not be of normal size and shape though the enamel is thinner than usual and may be pitted (Figure 1.3). These teeth are loosely attached to the gum tissue and have little or no root developed.

They may be a source of difficulty during feeding, especially for the mother in breast feeding, or a tongue ulcer may occur in the child from bottle feeding. Consequently in the past many of these teeth have been extracted. However, they are teeth of the normal series and if extracted no other primary teeth will take their place (Figure 1.4). Teeth that are allowed to remain in situ may not develop to their full potential, appearing discoloured (Figure 1.5).

Permanent Dentition

The first permanent teeth to come into the mouth or erupt are the first permanent molars which are positioned behind or distal to the second primary molar. Lower teeth tend to erupt before upper teeth at six years of age although there may be variation in this timing. At this age usually the lower central incisors are shed or exfoliate prior to the eruption of the central incisors (Figure 1.6).

The lower central incisors may come into the mouth spaced and symmetrically placed (Figure 1.7) or irregularly positioned and displaced (Figure 1.8). Marked

Figure 1.2. *Primary dentition.*

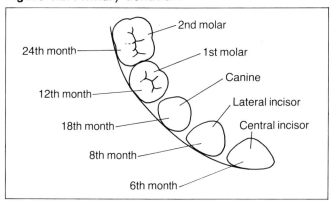

Figure 1.1. *Primary dentition of a child aged four years.*

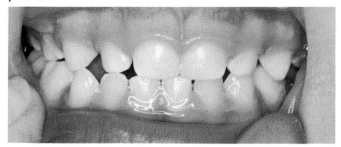

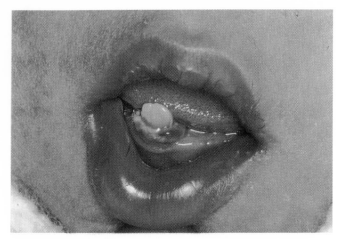

Figure 1.3. *Neonatal tooth in a child aged 10 days. Note the mild discoloration of the enamel and the swollen soft tissue at the point of attachment to the tooth.*

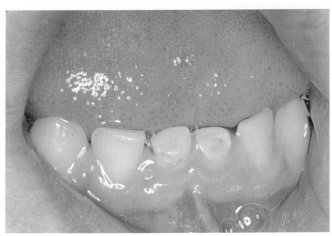

Figure 1.5. *Child aged three years who had retained neonatal central incisor teeth.*

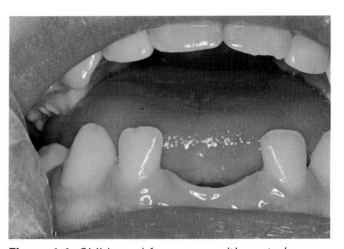

Figure 1.4. *Child aged four years with central incisors missing. Neonatal teeth were extracted during the neonatal period.*

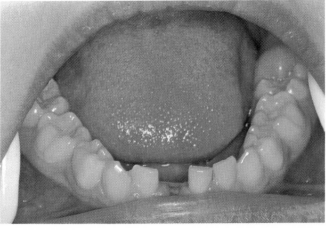

Figure 1.6. *Lower arch of a child aged six and a half years showing a nearly complete lower arch present. Note first permanent molars are erupting at this age and the right central incisor has been shed prior to the eruption of its successor.*

irregularity in the arrangement of the teeth is referred to as crowding and indicates a shortage of space for the teeth. Slight crowding may resolve or be acceptable, but crowding and irregularity affecting all the lower incisors (Figure 1.9) is a strong indication that treatment will be required at a later date. It is considered normal for the upper central incisors to erupt spaced one from the other (Figure 1.10) at eight years of age. The median space (between the central incisors) or diastema may be quite pronounced and not be eliminated until the lateral incisors come into position followed by the canines at 11 to 12 years. A median diastema in a child's dentition is often a cause of parental concern. Marked or severe anomalies of position of teeth

and their arrangement require the specialist advice of an orthodontist.

Anomalies in Number
Missing Teeth

The absence of one, several or all the teeth occurs in the primary and permanent dentitions. A major aetiological factor may be heredity, since a history of missing teeth may be traced through several generations of one family. Missing teeth represent a fault in the initiation or proliferation stage of a developing tooth. A diagnosis of complete or partial anodontia may be tentatively made when

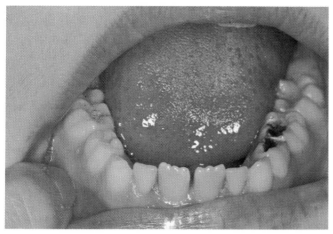

Figure 1.7. *Lower arch in a child aged seven years. Note erupted central incisors spaced and regularly positioned.*

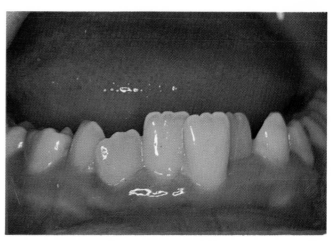

Figure 1.9. *Crowding of lower incisors.*

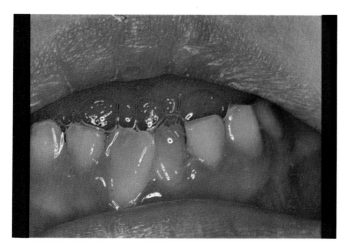

Figure 1.8. *Irregular positioning of central incisors.*

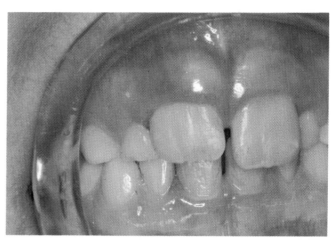

Figure 1.10. *Spacing between upper central incisors – median diastema. Normal development.*

teeth have not appeared nine months to a year after the usually expected time. Referral for confirmation of a provisional diagnosis is essential and diagnosis is easily confirmed by an intra-oral or extra-oral radiograph.

Missing teeth occur less frequently in the primary dentition and are relatively uncommon, the prevalence being one in 100 cases. Depending on the tooth or teeth in question treatment or artificial replacement may be necessary. Indications for a prosthesis are complete absence of the primary dentition, or if a group of teeth are missing, such that their absence may interfere with speech, masticatory function or cause a displeasing appearance (Figure 1.11).

The occurrence of missing teeth in the permanent dentition is more frequent. Prevalence figures of four to six per cent are often quoted. Excluding the third permanent molars, the tooth most commonly involved is the mandibular second premolar, followed by the upper lateral incisor. Often associated with partial anodontia is the presence of a 'peg-shaped' or cone-shaped lateral incisor (Figure 1.12).

Extra Teeth

The development of extra teeth above the normal number occurs in both dentitions but less commonly in the primary

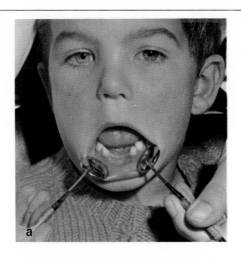

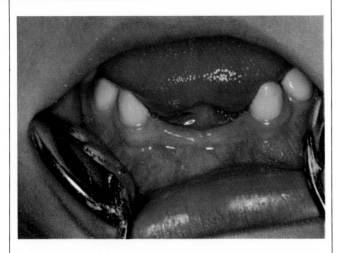

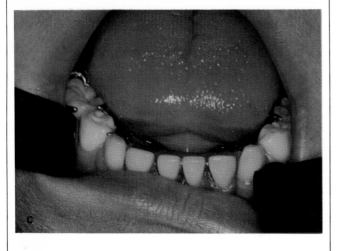

Figure 1.11. *(a) and (b) Missing primary lower incisors in a child aged four years. (c) Replacement of missing teeth by a partial denture to improve function and aesthetics.*

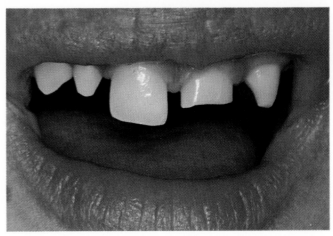

Figure 1.12. *Upper anterior teeth in the permanent dentition of a girl aged 11 years. The left lateral upper incisor is congenitally absent. The upper right lateral incisor is peg-shaped, and the neighbouring central incisor is coincidentally fractured.*

Figure 1.13. *Supernumerary erupted in the primary dentition palatal to the upper incisors.*

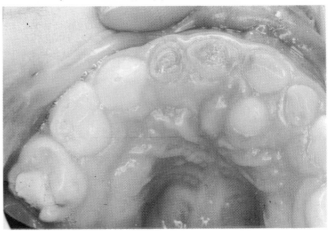

series. In this dentition the prevalence is quoted from 0.3 per cent to two per cent. Such teeth, termed supernumeraries, are usually found in the maxillary (Figure 1.13) or mandibular incisor regions.

Supernumerary teeth of the permanent dentition occur twice as frequently. The majority are found in the maxillary incisor region. One type, a mesiodens, occurs in the mid-line between the maxillary central incisors. Frequently such teeth are detected on radiographic examination during a routine check. Non-eruption of permanent maxillary incisors long after the normal time they are expected in the mouth should suggest the presence of a supernumerary which is interfering with the path of eruption of the incisor teeth (Figure 1.14). The diagnosis must be confirmed by radiography.

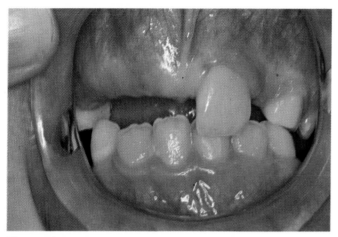

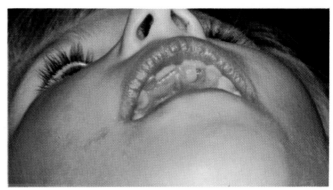

Figure 1.16. *Well defined cingulum on palatal aspect of upper left central incisor.*

Figure 1.14. *Non-eruption of central incisor due to presence of non-erupted supernumerary.*

Figure 1.17. *Primary and permanent teeth in the molar region showing the development of additional cusps.*

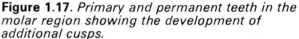

Figure 1.15. *Peg-shaped lower central incisors in the permanent dentition.*

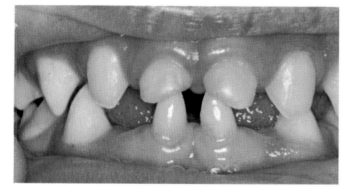

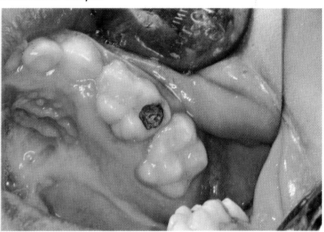

Figure 1.18. *Upper left lateral incisor shows three incisal tubercles which is normal of newly erupted teeth. Upper left central incisor demonstrates four such tubercles which is unusual but of no clinical significance.*

Anomalies of Shape

Developmental anomalies in the shape of teeth cover a wide range of conditions. A common example of variation in shape is the peg-shaped tooth. Such teeth may occur in other positions in the mouth although this is rare (Figure 1.15). A further variation in shape may be the presence of a pronounced cingulum (a prominence on the palatal aspect) usually associated with upper incisors (Figure 1.16). Treatment is indicated if this interferes with oral function, e.g. closing the mouth.

In addition, teeth may develop extra cusps; this is more common in the molar region (Figure 1.17) but may rarely manifest itself in a permanent central incisor (Figure 1.18). Incisor teeth normally have three tubercles on their incisal

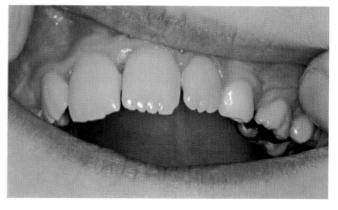

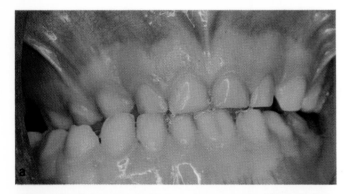

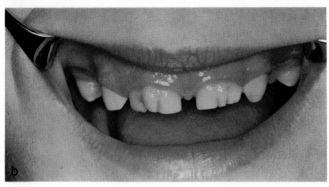

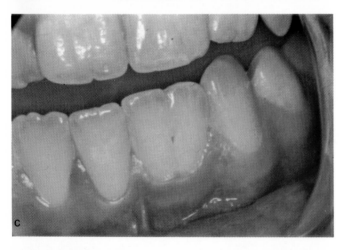

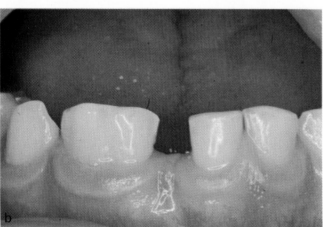

Figure 1.19. *(Left) (a) Gemination (twinning) of the lower left primary lateral incisor. (b) Gemination of the upper right primary central incisor. Fusion of the left incisors. (c) Fusion of the lower left permanent incisors. (d) Fusion of the lower right primary incisors.*

edge. These tend to be worn away by attrition.

An apparent increase in the size of the crown of a tooth may be due to gemination or twinning. Such teeth are said to develop from one tooth germ and have one root canal although two crowns develop side by side and may be joined at any point along their length. Gemination may be confirmed by radiographic examination and by the fact that there are the correct number of teeth present or developing (Figure 1.19, a and b). Similar in clinical appearance but of a different cause is fusion, where two neighbouring teeth are joined by their calcified tissues. Again identification of the teeth present or developing in the jaws will aid diagnosis (Figure 1.19, b, c and d). Treatment may or may not be required but continual observation of the line of gemination or fusion of the enamel is necessary, as often this is a susceptible area for a carious attack.

Anomalies of Structure
Inherited Syndromes

In general terms there are two major groups. First, hereditary syndromes which include amelogenesis imperfecta (a developmental defect in enamel) and dentinogenesis imperfecta (a developmental defect in dentine) and, second, non-inherited conditions such as the hypoplasias of the calcified tooth tissues due to premature birth, and neonatal factors or febrile diseases. There are many less common aetiological factors in the second group. The overall incidence of amelogenesis imperfecta is reported as one in 14,000. There are different types of the condition, some are grouped as hereditary enamel hypoplasias and others as hereditary hypocalcifications.

Clinically the hypoplasias may appear as smaller teeth with a hard smooth surface—yellow to orange-brown in colour (Figure 1.20), or teeth of normal size and a relatively normal colour but with either pitted or wrinkled enamel. The enamel of teeth in the hypocalcification group tends to be softer than normal enamel, their colour may vary from yellow to grey-brown to dull white. Dental advice should be sought if such conditions are suspected or if it is known that other family members have had any of these conditions. Early treatment by crowning of the teeth may be strongly indicated if a functional dentition is to be maintained and to improve appearance.

Dentinogenesis imperfecta (hereditary opalescent

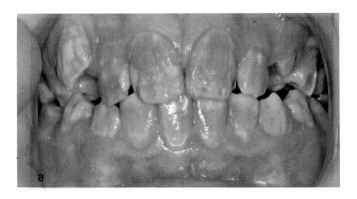 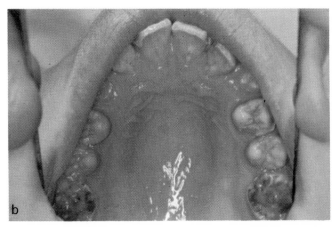

Figure 1.20. *(a) and (b) Two examples of amelogenesis imperfecta affecting the permanent dentition.*

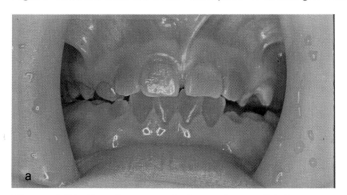 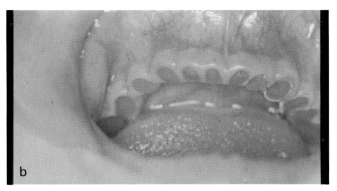

Figure 1.21. *Dentinogenesis imperfecta of (a) permanent dentition and (b) primary dentition. The teeth are worn down to the gum margin.*

Figure 1.22. *(a) and (b) Enamel hypoplasia following a series of systemic diseases during the first year and a half of life. Note the incisors and first permanent molars are markedly affected.*

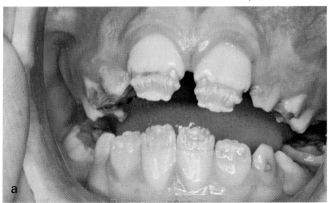 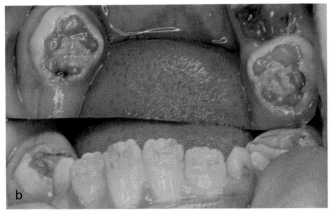

dentine) has an incidence of one in 8,000. It is a simple, dominant non sex-linked condition affecting the dentine of all the teeth. Clinically, the teeth are blue-grey to brown in colour and may have an opalescent appearance (Figure 1.21a). The dentino-enamel junction tends to be physically weak and thus the overlying enamel is quickly abraded. Teeth in such cases are often worn down to the gum margin before being referred for treatment (Figure 1.21b).

Non-inherited Syndromes

Of the non-genetic hypoplasias those related to febrile or systemic diseases are the most common and very disfiguring. Usually those parts of the teeth that are undergoing formation at the time of the illness may be involved. Severe illnesses experienced during the first years of life are recorded as kymographic records on the incisal por-

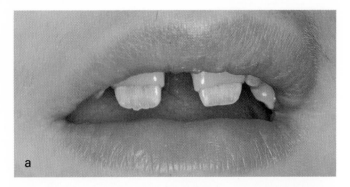

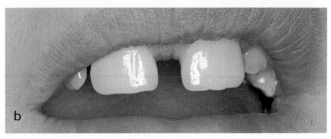

Figure 1.23. *(a) The incisal tips of the upper central incisors are hypoplastic following systemic disease during the first year of life. (b) Aesthetic improvement following crowning.*

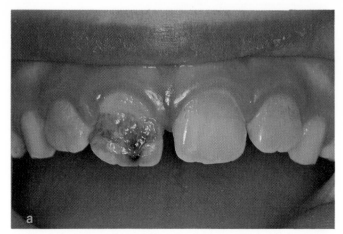

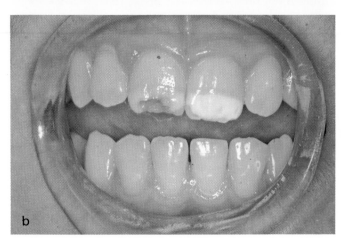

Figure 1.25. *(a) and (b) Localized enamel hypoplasia of upper central incisors. Note remaining teeth are unaffected.*

Figure 1.24. *(a) Hypoplasia of the upper anterior teeth following illness in childhood. (b) Improvement of aesthetics following crowning of the upper incisors.*

Figure 1.26. *Tetracycline staining of the teeth of the primary dentition.*

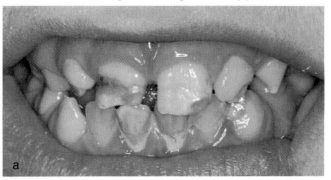

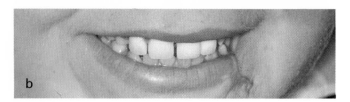

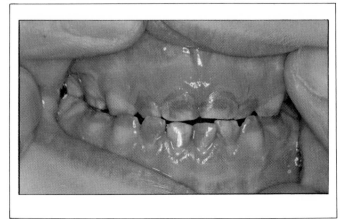

tions of the anterior teeth (Figure 1.22, a and b). However, it may be difficult to pin-point a cause and effect relationship, since a history of such illnesses is almost invariably retrospective. Hypoplasias of teeth in young children can be a cause of great distress due to the unsightly appearance. It is nearly always possible to carry out quite sophisticated crowning of such teeth with a great improvement in the appearance and subsequent happiness of the child (Figures 1.23 and 1.24).

On occasion local factors such as a dental infection from a primary tooth may affect a permanent successor, or a blow to a developing tooth may cause a hypoplastic defect to an individual tooth or a pair of neighbouring teeth (Figure 1.25).

Anomalies in Colour

Tetracyclines chelate with calcium ions and therefore are built in with teeth or bones forming at the time the drug is taken. The effect on the tooth enamel is permanent. It is not uncommon to see discoloured primary (Figure 1.26) and permanent teeth due to tetracycline drug therapy. Depending on the type of drug administered the resulting colour may be grey-brown, yellow or brownish-yellow. A marked degree of discoloration may require the patient to be fitted with crowns for the upper permanent incisors. Practitioners should, wherever possible and where there is a choice of drugs available, avoid prescribing tetracyclines for expectant mothers and children.

2. The Jaws

G. R. Seward and D. A. McGowan

The jaws and dental arches make up the middle and lower thirds of the skeleton of the face and so their shape, size and relationship have a fundamental effect on facial form. There is an undoubted popular tendency to regard certain types of facial appearance as indicating qualities of character—the 'lantern-jawed' tough as opposed to the 'chinless wonder' for example. The unfortunate adolescent with protruding teeth, if a boy, may be dismissed as being stupid or, if a girl, described as 'horsey'.

Facial Deformities

Facial deformity is a relative term, bearing in mind the wide range of socially acceptable facial patterns. However, gross discrepancies in the size and shape of the upper and lower jaws may produce a facial appearance which the patient feels is unacceptable, and such self-consciousness of appearance may verge on psychiatric disorder at times.

Patients and, indeed, their medical advisors, are often unaware of the help that specialist oral surgeons can offer. The operations are technically complex and the post-operative period, which usually involves a period of jaw immobilization, is uncomfortable. Such treatment, therefore, is never undertaken without the patient's full knowledge of the complications and his unreserved consent. The four main types of deformity are:

1. Relative protrusion of the mandible (Figure 2.1).

2. Relative protrusion of the maxilla (Figures 2.2 and 2.3).

3. 'Open bite'—where the anterior teeth do not meet (Figure 2.4).

4. Asymmetry of the mandible (Figure 2.5).

In many cases more than one element is abnormal and there may be compensating changes in the adjacent tissues in response to the basic defect.

Examination of the relationship of the incisor teeth with the jaws closed together will help to identify the basic abnormality. The patient must be told to 'close on your back teeth', otherwise a forward posturing of the mandible may bring the teeth into a misleading 'edge to edge' relation. Detailed diagnosis depends upon the analysis of special x-rays taken with a cephalostat—a positioning device for ensuring direct comparability of films of different patients, or the same patient at different times. Such films and tracings from them are used, along with casts of the dentition, for the detailed planning of the corrective surgery. Less major variations from the normal can be treated by altering the position of the teeth by orthodontic methods, and this will be discussed later.

Aetiology

Quite commonly the condition is inherited and patients may seek treatment even against the advice of their parents, who being similarly affected, regard such facial appearance as normal! Old family photographs may be of interest in this context. The portraits of the Royal House of Hapsburg illustrate generations of mandibular prognathism and this particular deformity is still sometimes known as the 'Hapsburg jaw'.

Inadequately treated fractures of the facial bones or severe infection of the jaws in childhood may also be a cause of facial deformity, but such cases are rarely seen nowadays in Britain. Apart from frank neoplasia of the jaws with consequent swelling, hyperplasia of the mandibular condyle may give rise to asymmetry of the mandible (Figure 2.5). Ankylosis of the mandible is a most disabling condition and surgical treatment is almost always necessary.

Treatment

Jaw deformity usually becomes noticeable during the adolescent growth period when all the permanent teeth except the third molars have erupted, but corrective surgery is often postponed until jaw growth is complete. A patient's distress about his appearance at this sensitive age may,

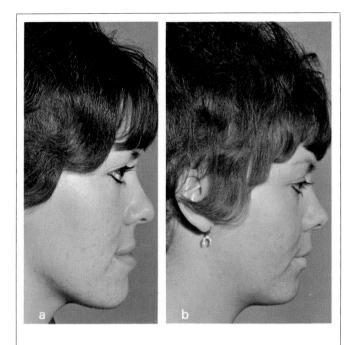

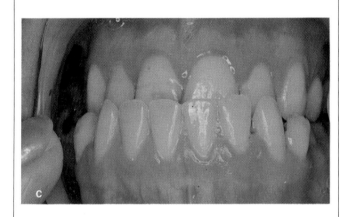

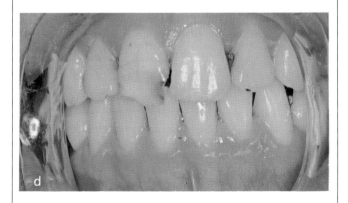

Figure 2.1. *For details see text.*

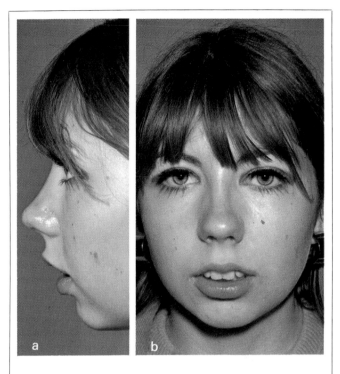

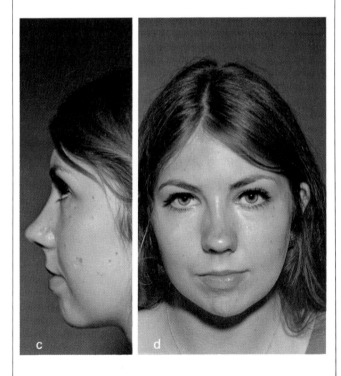

Figure 2.2. *For details see text.*

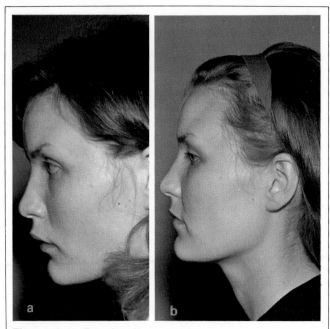

Figure 2.3. *For details see text.*

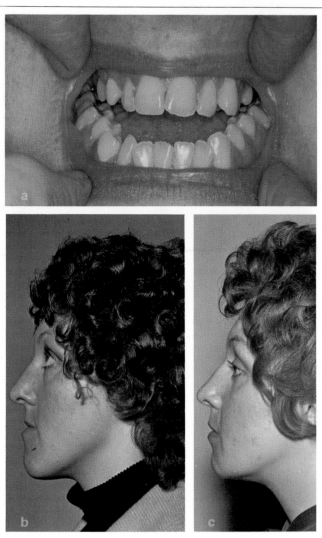

Figure 2.4. *For details see text.*

however, persuade the surgeon to operate without delay. Most cases are treated with the cooperation of an orthodontist who can improve tooth position by means of appliances on the basis of the new jaw relationship created surgically.

A wide range of operative techniques for correction of jaw deformity have been developed. One of the most versatile is that developed by Professor Obwegeser of Zurich (Figure 2.6). The operation is performed via an intra-oral approach so that no skin incision is necessary. The ascending ramus of the mandible on each side is exposed and the attached muscles stripped off. A horizontal cut is made with a drill above the level of the mandibular foramen through the lingual cortical plate. A vertical cut is made in the lower molar region through the buccal cortical plate. These two cuts are joined by a third made along the anterior edge of the ramus. Two osteotomes are inserted into this cut and by judicious leverage the ramus is split in the sagittal plane. This allows the jaws to be placed in the new relationship as judged by the interdigitation of the teeth. The mandibular fragments are then held together in the new position by wire ligatures and the soft tissues are closed with sutures. The jaws are immobilized in the new relationship—usually by metal cap splints—for four to six weeks, by which time bony union at the operation site should be present. This procedure can be applied to the correction of suitable cases of any of the four main types of deformity.

Clinical Examples
Protrusion of the Mandible

Patient 1 (Figure 2.1) had her lower jaw protrusion reduced by this operation. The improvement in her profile is shown (b) and also the change in relationship of her teeth (c and d). It should be noted that the unsightly upper right central incisor has since been crowned. Such treatment has to be postponed until a stable jaw relationship is achieved.

Protrusion of the Maxilla

Patient 2 (Figure 2.2) had the reverse problem. Due to retrusion of the mandible, her upper incisors appeared to

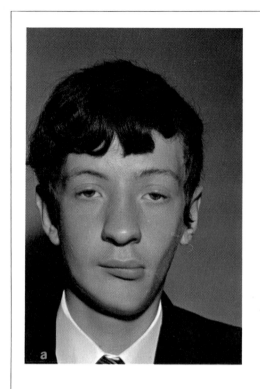

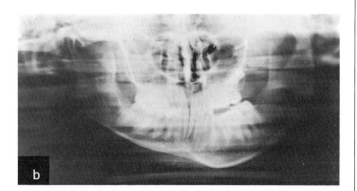

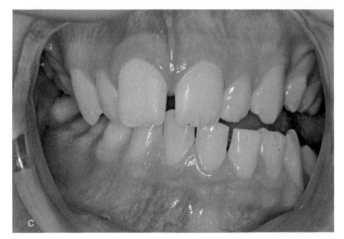

Figure 2.5. *For details see text.*

Figure 2.6 *The horizontal cut AB on the lingual side (1) is joined to the vertical cut CD on the buccal side (2) by the intermediate cut BC. The ramus and angle are split (3). The hatched portion of the bone is removed to allow a mortise joint, when backward movement of the tooth-bearing fragment is required (4). Forward movement of rotation may be achieved (5 and 6).*

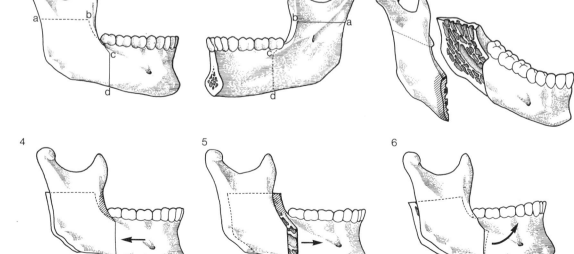

be unduly prominent and prevented closure of her lips (a and b). This situation was relieved by the same sagittal splitting operation as in the previous case, but this time with forward movement of the mandible. After operation the relevant prominence of the upper incisors is reduced and the lips are easily closed at rest (c and d).

Patient 3 had an apparently similar problem (Figure 2.3) but in this case correction was achieved by operation on the maxilla alone since it was felt that this was where the basic defect lay. Again a marked improvement was achieved (Figure 2.3b).

Anterior Open Bite

Patient 4 presented basically as an 'open bite' problem (Figure 2.4a) but an element of relative maxillary retrusion was also present (b). Correction was achieved by repositioning the maxillary segment en bloc—the line of section passing just above the level of the roots of the upper teeth through the maxillary antra and the floor of the nose. Section of the anterior part of the mandible on both sides with an upwards and posterior movement of the incisor

segment was carried out simultaneously. The post-operative profile is shown (c).

Asymmetry of the Mandible

Patient 5 has a gross asymmetry of his mandible due to condylar hyperplasia (Figure 2.5). The shape of the jaw is well demonstrated by a special radiographic technique (rotational tomography, b). The abnormality of his incisor relationship is immediately apparent (c). This young man's treatment so far has been by orthodontic and prosthetic methods and has been directed to prevention of compensatory changes. Surgical treatment is envisaged once growth has ceased.

Conclusion

Surgical correction has a lot to offer to patients with facial deformity or disharmony. The apparent change in personality after operation is usually quite dramatic. Indeed the appearance of an engagement ring on the finger of a young woman after operation is held by many oral surgeons to be the best indicator of a successful result!

3. The Tongue, Tori and Fordyce Spots

C. E. Renson

Developmental defects of the tongue are rare but they do occur and may be associated with heart disease.

Median Rhomboid Glossitis

This appears clinically as an ovoid, diamond, or rhomboid-shaped reddish patch on the dorsal surface immediately anterior to the circumvallate papillae (Figure 3.1). The patch is devoid of filiform papillae. The lesion is not inflammatory in origin, as its name implies, but is due to the failure of the tuberculum impar to retract before fusion of the lateral prominences of the tongue. The condition is most obvious clinically, when the tongue is heavily coated. Until recently median rhomboid glossitis was thought to be a congenital defect which remained undiscovered until adult life. However, recent work by Cooke (1975) appears to incriminate *Candida albicans*. Invasion by the fungus over a period of years may result in the characteristic appearance of median rhomboid glossitis. It is occasionally mistaken for carcinoma, which is extremely rare in this location. The incidence is said to be less than one per cent.

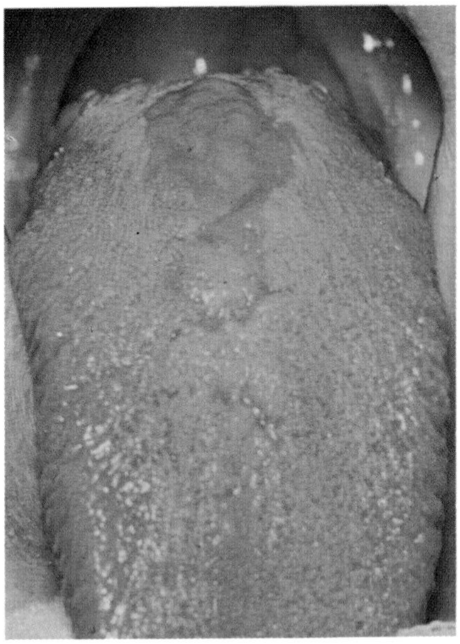

Figure 3.1. *Median rhomboid glossitis.*

Fissured Tongue

This is also termed scrotal, furrowed or grooved tongue and may be congenital or acquired (Figure 3.2). Numerous small furrows or grooves are present on the dorsum of the tongue, frequently they radiate from a deep median groove. A mild glossitis may occasionally result from the trapping of bacteria and food debris in the deeper grooves. Stretching and flattening the fissures and using a toothbrush on gauze to cleanse the surface is usually the only treatment necessary. The rate of incidence has not been determined since there is disagreement as to what constitutes a fissured tongue.

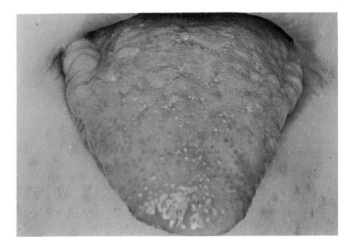

Figure 3.2. *(Right) Scrotal tongue.*

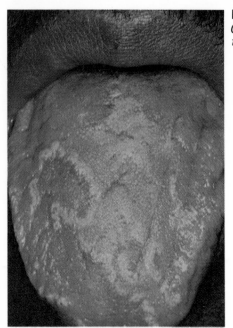

Figure 3.3.
Geographic tongue.

Geographic Tongue (Erythema Migrans Linguae)

Here the tongue exhibits smooth red patches where the filiform papillae have been lost (Figure 3.3). The patches, which have a greyish-yellow elevated border, are of an irregular pattern. This is not a true developmental defect but usually starts in childhood and may persist throughout life, or disappear in middle age. The aetiology of the condition is not known although various workers have detected a heredity factor and also associations with rickets and fissured tongue. The areas of desquamation remain for a short time in one location and then heal and appear in another location, giving rise to the condition's descriptive name. There may be periods when the tongue is completely healed. The condition may persist for many years and there is no satisfactory treatment. It causes no physical discomfort but patients may need continual reassurance of its innocuousness.

Hairy Tongue

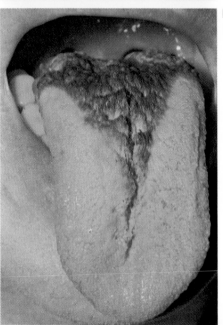

Figure 3.4.
Hairy tongue.

Not a true developmental defect but it is best considered with tongue conditions in this group (Figure 3.4). Here the filiform papillae of an area of the dorsum hypertrophy, and normal desquamation ceases. As a result, the elongated papillae form a matted layer which may be yellowish-white to brown, or even black in colour. Extrinsic staining of the 'hairs' by food, tobacco or chromogenic bacteria usually occurs. The condition has been observed at all ages and the aetiology remains unknown although various workers have implicated fungi, systemic disturbances, such as anaemia or gastric upsets, or the oral consumption of drugs, such as sodium perborate, sodium peroxide, penicillin, etc. It has also been noted as a finding following irradiation about the head and neck in the treatment of a malignant growth.

Apart from the alarming appearance, some patients may complain of retching or gagging and of the tongue sticking to the palate on waking. Brushing the tongue with a toothbrush promotes desquamation and removes debris. Tablets containing 100 mg ascorbic acid, 70 mg sodium percarbonate and 0.2 mg copper sulphate dissolved in a small volume of water and brushed onto the surface of the tongue are helpful in relieving the condition.

Ankyloglossia or 'Tongue Tie'

This condition occurs when an abnormally short lingual fraenum is present, or when the fraenum is attached near the tongue tip. Speech difficulties and inability to protrude

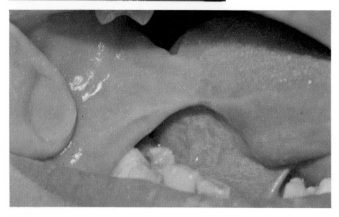

Figure 3.5. *(Left) Tongue tie. The tongue is attached to the cheek.*

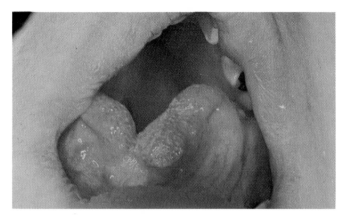

Figure 3.6. *Bifid tongue.*

Figure 3.7. *Fordyce spots.*

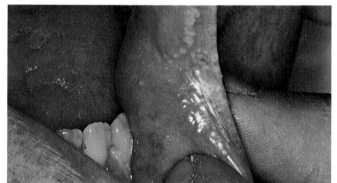

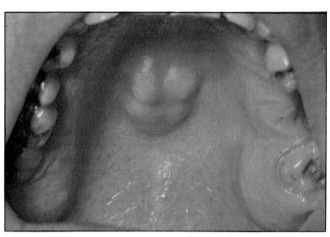

Figure 3.8. *A mid-line exostosis of the hard palate: torus palatinus.*

Figure 3.9. *Two mandibular exostoses: torus mandibularis.*

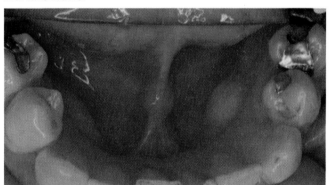

the tongue usually result in early detection of this defect. In infants the fraenum may be snipped with scissors; in adults it usually has to be dissected out. Although the offending fraenum is usually centrally placed, occasionally ankyloglossia can be caused by an attachment between the mucosa lining the cheek and the lateral border of the tongue (Figure 3.5).

Bifid Tongue

A completely bifid tongue is a rare condition which is apparently due to the failure of the two lateral halves of the tongue to fuse in the mid-line. A partially cleft tongue is more common and manifests as a deep groove in the dorsum. It is of little clinical significance except that food debris, which tends to collect in the cleft base, may give rise to a glossitis. In Figure 3.6 the bifid tongue was associated with a cleft palate. The tag of tissue situated in the bifurcation is muscle apparently formed in an effort to obliterate the defect.

Fordyce Spots

Sometimes known as Fordyce's granules or Fordyce's disease, the condition was originally described by Fordyce in 1896 as occurring on the lips and buccal mucosa. Figure 3.7 illustrates the typical appearance of these small, light yellow macular areas when they occur on the lips. They are ectopic sebaceous glands and occur in about 80 per cent of the population. They are found most commonly in the buccal mucosa, the retromolar region and the lips, but can occur in the gingiva and palate. They may appear as small yellow spots or may form relatively large yellow patches which project slightly above the surface of the surrounding tissue. Fewer children than adults exhibit Fordyce spots, because although they may be present they usually remain small and undeveloped until puberty. However, they have been reported long before puberty. These ectopic glands cause no discomfort, have no clinical or functional significance and require no treatment.

Developmental Defects of the Mouth and Jaws

Oral Tori

The oral tori are exostoses, i.e. localized peripheral overgrowths of bone which are continuous with the original bone.

Torus Palatinus

This is an exostosis occurring in the mid-line of the hard palate. Figure 3.8 illustrates a torus palatinus of the lobular type with a well-defined mid-line groove. Various sizes and shapes occur, from a small flat elevation to a large nodular mass. The torus can be regarded as a continuation of growth of margins of the palatine processes. The cause is unknown but evidence has been offered that tori are hereditary conditions, thought to follow a mendelian dominant pattern. The estimated incidence is about 20 to 25 per cent. Women are more often affected than men, and most cases are not observed before the age of 30 years. The overlying mucosa occasionally appears blanched and may become ulcerated if traumatized. In slight cases no treatment is indicated. If the torus is large and causing discomfort, or if it interferes with a denture fitting, it should be surgically removed.

Torus Mandibularis

This is an exostosis which usually occurs bilaterally on the lingual aspect of the mandible opposite the canine and premolar teeth (see Figure 3.9). Like the palatine torus it can vary considerably in size and shape. The cause is unknown, but the condition is thought to be inherited. It has been noted that the exostosis occurs at the site of the junction of two different methods of ossification, Meckel's cartilage and membranous covering. The incidence is about seven per cent, and the condition does not usually become noticeable until the third decade. Treatment is indicated if difficulty is experienced in fitting a lower denture.

Cooke, B. E. D., *Br. J. Derm.,* 1975, **93**, 399.

Section 2
Diseases of the Teeth and Supporting Structures

4. Caries and Pulp Disease

D. S. Berman and C. E. Renson

Dental caries is the most frequently occurring disease of the dental and oral tissues. On average by the age of five years, children will have at least four or five teeth affected by the disease. By 15 years as many as 10 permanent teeth may be decayed, missing or filled as a result of carious involvement. The relative importance of the disease, however, is not only the severity of the destructive processes, although these can be extremely harmful, but that it attacks nearly all the population, thereby creating a major public health problem besides much discomfort for the individual.

Essentially dental caries is a disease of the calcified tissues of the teeth. It is a progressively destructive process initiated by bacterial activity in the presence of a suitable substrate (e.g. sucrose). It occurs on the outer surfaces of the teeth at sites of predilection and progresses inwards towards the centre of the tooth, the dental pulp. The bacteria are localized at the point of attack in a material called bacterial (or dental) plaque. Bacterial plaque is an adherent film of infected mucinous material. It forms continuously and is not easily removed.

Caries

Common Sites of Attack

One of the common sites for the carious process to begin is the occlusal or biting surfaces of the molars and premolars. This is mainly due to the presence of fissures which encourage food retention. Figure 4.1 demonstrates the retention of chocolate in the occlusal pattern of upper first molars and premolars of the permanent dentition. The presence of such cariogenic food encourages the production of acid by the action of oral bacteria. The initial effect on the teeth may go undetected for some time, the first visible changes being discoloration of the deepest parts of the occlusal surfaces, the fissures. Such discoloration or staining is seen on the biting surfaces of the lower molar teeth in Figure 4.2. This additionally shows a

Figure 4.2. *Discoloration of the fissures of the occlusal surfaces of lower first permanent molars. There has been loss of occlusal enamel, due to involvement by caries of the underlying tooth structure.*

Figure 4.1. *Chocolate retained on the biting (occlusal) surfaces of an upper first molar and premolars of the permanent dentition.*

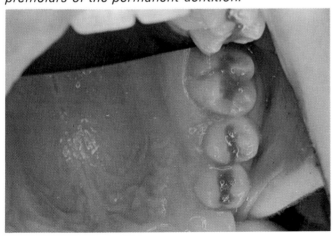

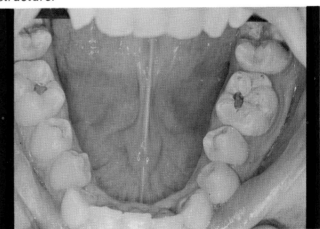

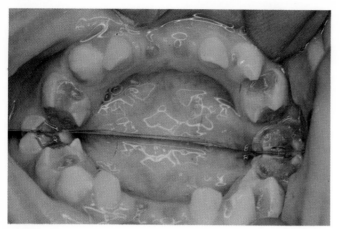

Figure 4.3. *Lower primary teeth viewed in a mirror. The molars show excessive tooth loss due to the carious process.*

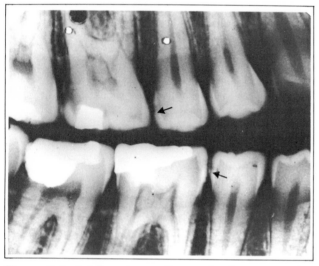

Figure 4.4. *A bite-wing radiograph of upper and lower teeth. Radiolucent areas are shown (arrowed) on the distal surfaces of the upper and lower second premolars, where they contact the first permanent molars. These represent carious lesions which were not detectable clinically by visual examination.*

Figure 4.5. *Carious lesions at the necks of the teeth (cervical margins) near the gum margins. This site of carious attack occurs more commonly in older people.*

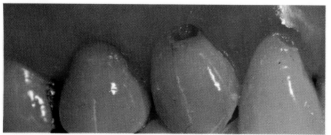

small dark area where the occlusal enamel has been lost. At this stage the disease process has involved a larger portion of the body of the tooth (including the dentine) than is apparent by external examination. Eventual destruction of the dentine will cause the overlying enamel to be unsupported with its eventual collapse (Figure 4.3).

The areas where neighbouring teeth come into contact (the contact areas) are common sites for caries to develop. These tooth surfaces of contiguous teeth are termed the 'approximal' surfaces and encourage the retention of bacterial plaque. Unfortunately the early detection of the disease at these sites is extremely difficult, even by a dental surgeon, using normal visual diagnostic aids. It is for the diagnosis of 'approximal caries' that intra-oral radiography (bite-wing radiographs) is used. By passing x-rays through the contact areas of teeth dental decay is shown as a radiolucent area. Figure 4.4 shows a bite-wing radiograph of an adult. The upper and lower second premolars show approximal lesions which were not detectable by visual examination. The important point is that on examining teeth that appear healthy in the mouth, approximal lesions may be present that will only show on a radiograph. Therefore, regular checks with the dentist for early diagnosis are essential.

The necks of the teeth at the gum margin are a third site of attack. This occurs more commonly in older people (Figure 4.5); an attack of sudden onset may be associated with constant sweet sucking following the abandonment of smoking.

Acute Caries

Distinction is often made between active and quiescent phases of the caries attack. Active or acute caries is a rapid process and may easily involve the dental pulp before the tooth has had a chance to protect itself. It is more commonly seen in the mouths of young children. Figure 4.6a shows the destroyed approximal surface of a lower primary molar. The light yellow colour is typical of an acute attack. A section cut from the centre of the tooth (Figure 4.6b) shows a great deal of destruction of the calcified tissues and appears to have reached the central chamber of the tooth where the nerve or pulp is located. This is confirmed in Figure 4.6c, which is a decalcified section of the same tooth and shows evidence of a pulpal abscess in the pulp cavity. In fact this tooth was extracted from a very young child because of toothache.

Chronic Caries

By contrast, Figure 4.7a illustrates arrested or chronic caries in an upper primary molar of a young child. A large portion of the occlusal and approximal enamel and dentine has been destroyed. The superficial decayed dentine is

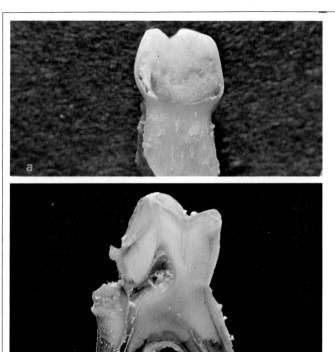

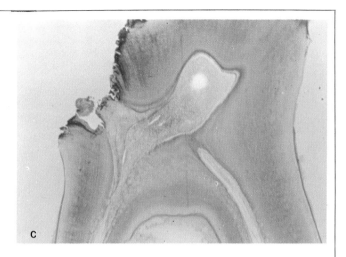

Figure 4.6. *(a) Extracted lower first primary molar. The approximal and part of the occlusal surface is severely destroyed by caries. The light yellow colour indicates a rapid involvement (acute attack) of the tooth tissue. (b) A vertical ground section cut from the same tooth showing severe destruction of the tooth. The carious process has even extended to the pulp chamber. (c) A vertical decalcified and stained section of the same tooth. There is an abscess in the pulp cavity.*

Figure 4.7. *(a) An upper second primary molar with an occlusal and approximal carious lesion. The dark discoloration of the superficial layer of caries suggests a slower or arrested caries process. (b) A vertical ground section of the same tooth. There is the superficial dark layer of carious dentine with an underlying dark blue band (translucent zone). This represents a reaction of the tooth to slow down or prevent the passage of toxins or bacteria towards the pulp. (c) A vertical decalcified and stained section of the same tooth. There has been penetration of the dentine by bacteria. At the periphery of the pulp chamber and below the carious dentine, a calcified barrier (reparative dentine) has been formed by the dental pulp. This is a further defence reaction by the tooth.*

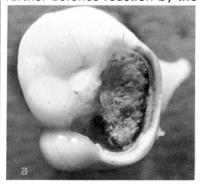

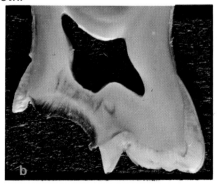

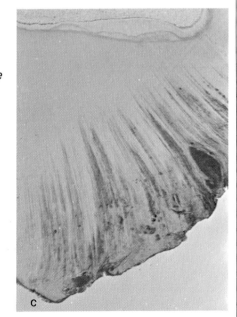

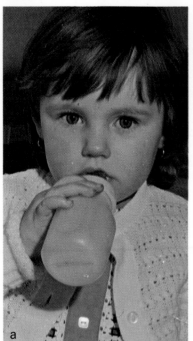

Figure 4.8. *(a) Child sucking sweetened orange juice from a bottle. Continuous imbibing through the day or night can have a marked deleterious effect on the teeth of young children. (b) The upper anterior primary teeth of the same child. The teeth have been subject to an attack of rampant caries.*

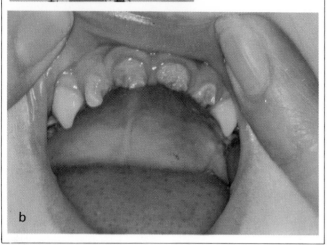

Figure 4.9. *Arrested caries of the upper anterior primary teeth of a young child.*

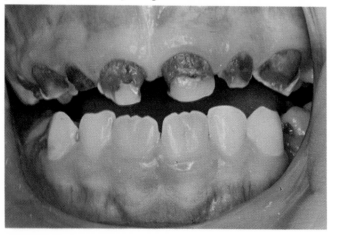

coloured dark brown and is typical of arrested caries. A section through the tooth and lesion (Figure 4.7b) shows a defence reaction on the part of the remaining vital tooth. The dark blue band below the superficial brown area is a 'translucent zone' and represents the formation of a calcified barrier which prevents or slows down the passage of toxins or bacteria towards the pulp. The presence of bacteria is denoted in Figure 4.7c by the areas which are stained dark blue. Of significance, however, is the presence of a second defence barrier at the periphery of the pulp. This has been formed in response to the dental caries attack. Therefore, even though teeth may show severe destruction, they may still protect themselves and, with the aid of dental treatment to seal off the infected area, may not require extraction.

Rampant Caries

This is a form of acute caries and is characterized by being a very rapid and burrowing process of sudden onset. A further feature being the attack of tooth surfaces which are normally considered relatively resistant to carious attack. It is not uncommon. A major aetiological factor is the retention of sweet, sticky substances on the tooth surfaces. An important vehicle for these substances are sweetened comforters. Children who imbibe sweetened fruit and vitamin juices through a bottle comforter, such as the child in Figure 4.8a, nearly always end up as she

Figure 4.10. *(a) Patient exhibiting swelling of left cheek, dental abscess of upper left lateral incisor. (b) Apical bone resorption due to infected pulp. (c) Pus draining from opening into pulp chamber. (d) Swelling has subsided following drainage. (e) Root canal filling in situ. (f) Resolution of area above root in (e). New bone has been formed.*

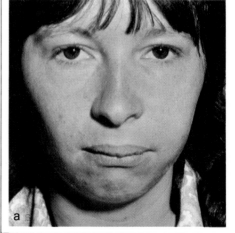

22

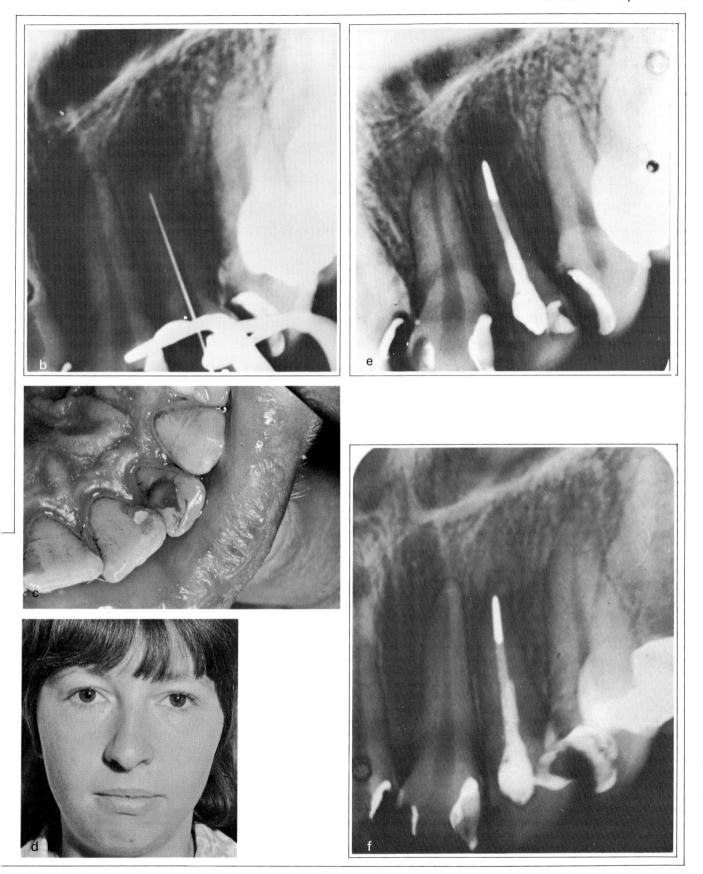

appears in Figure 4.8b. The severe destruction of the upper primary incisors is readily seen even in this very young child. The same effect may be produced by the prolonged use of a bottle at night containing milk and sugar, long after the normal weaning time. The onset of such a condition is insidious and is first seen as a white line of enamel decalcification at the gum margins of the teeth. In adults, when smoking is abandoned, sweet sucking (often peppermints) replaces the smoking habit with the same disastrous results. Referral for dietary advice is imperative in such situations. Although often the process is too far advanced for restoration of the anterior teeth in the young child, by the institution of preventive measures, the active lesions may become arrested as shown in Figure 4.9.

Treatment and Sequelae

Dental caries can, to a large extent, be prevented through fluoridation of the water supply, control of frequency of dietary sugar intake, and by the use of measures by the dentist (including the topical application of fluorides). However, once the disease has occurred its effect may be limited (secondary prevention) by correct dental treat-ment. Even a tooth with an infected pulp chamber may be conserved on occasion. The patient in Figure 4.10a was suffering from an acute abscess of the upper left second incisor. The pulp was infected and bone resorption had occurred at the tip of the root (Figure 4.10b). Pus was drained from the tooth via a hole on the palatal aspect (Figure 4.10c), thus converting the acute phase into a chronic one. The patient experienced immediate relief (Figure 4.10d). Subsequently the pulp canal was rendered infection free and was obliterated with filling material (Figure 4.10e). The radiograph taken four months later (Figure 4.10f) shows complete resolution with new bone laid down at the root apex.

Conclusion

It has been shown that dental caries can be prevented, is treatable when it occurs, particularly if detected at an early stage, and that measures can be taken to prevent its recurrence.

Further Reading
Silverstone, Leon M., *Preventive Dentistry*, Update, London, 1978

5. Periodontal Disease

J. Lozdan

The Normal Periodontium

The periodontium is defined as the supporting structures of the tooth and includes the gingiva (gum), periodontal membrane, alveolar bone and the cementum (Figure 5.1). The only part of the periodontium which is visible under normal circumstances is the gum, which is bounded by the gingival margin above and by the muco-gingival line or junction below and is divided clinically into papillary, marginal and attached areas. In health (Figure 5.2) the gum is scalloped in outline, has a knife edge margin where it meets the tooth, is often stippled and can vary in colour from coral pink to brown, black or blue depending on the degree of individual pigmentation. This should therefore be taken into account before making a diagnosis of Addison's disease or other disturbances of pigmentation. The narrow space between the gum and the tooth is known as the gingival crevice and varies in depth when healthy from between 0 to 2 mm. When the teeth are fully erupted the gingival margin is situated under the maximum convexity of the tooth at the cement–enamel junction (neck or cervical portion).

Chronic Periodontitis (Pyorrhea, Gingivitis)

Chronic inflammation is the most common disease process to affect the periodontium, and is the major factor responsible for tooth loss in adults. The disease is prevalent in most countries of the world, including the UK where a recent government survey has shown that about 30 million people are affected. It is a slow insidious process which begins in childhood and only becomes evident to the patient much later in life, by which time most of the supporting structures have been lost and the teeth have to be extracted. Contrary to popular belief chronic periodontitis is preventable, and if established is treatable, so that the days when a patient's dentition was condemned because of pyorrhea are over. In this day and age with

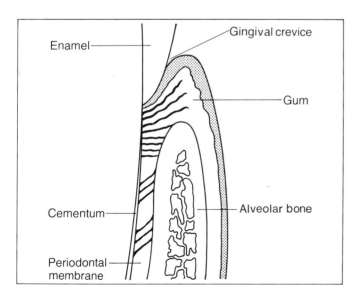

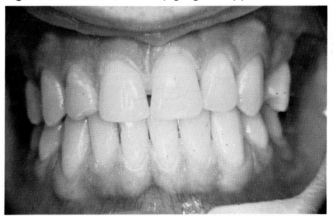

Figure 5.1. *(Left) The structures which form the periodontium.*

Figure 5.2. *(Below) Healthy gingival appearance.*

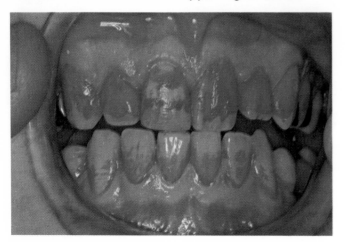

Figure 5.3. *Bacterial dental plaque disclosed by erythrosin dye.*

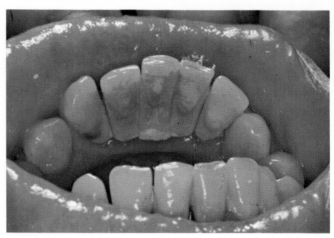

Figure 5.4. *Calculus on lingual surfaces of lower incisors.*

proper treatment patients should be able to retain their own natural teeth throughout life.

Bacterial Dental Plaque

The main aetiological factor responsible for chronic periodontitis is bacterial dental plaque, an extremely thin, tenacious, adherent mucinous film which forms on the surface of the tooth close to the gingival margin (Figure 5.3). Plaque consists of a mucoprotein matrix, derived from saliva, in which colonies of millions of organisms are embedded. It is the products of these organisms, i.e. enzymes, toxins and cell wall antigens, which are primarily responsible for the disease. The chronic nature of the disease is related to the persistent nature of plaque which can only be removed by dentist or patient or both.

Calculus (Tartar)

When plaque calcifies it is known as calculus or tartar and can vary in colour from light brown to black (Figure 5.4). It can be situated supra- or subgingivally and must be removed by instrumentation, as it is extremely hard and has a chemical composition similar to that of bone. Calculus always has a layer of soft plaque on its surface, and it is this factor which implicates it in the aetiology of the disease. Badly designed and constructed restorations and dental appliances are aggravating factors as they facilitate the accumulation of plaque which is then inaccessible to routine methods of removal, such as toothbrushing.

Signs, Symptoms and Treatment of Chronic Periodontitis

Bleeding from the gums. Bleeding from the gums after eating or toothbrushing may be one of the earliest signs and symptoms of chronic periodontitis. Unfortunately, it is regarded by most patients as a normal event which will follow the overzealous use of a toothbrush. This is a fallacy which needs to be dispelled. Healthy gums very rarely bleed. Haemorrhage results from trauma (e.g. toothbrushing) to the fragile vessels in inflamed tissues. The treatment is simple, and involves the removal of bacterial plaque which is followed by the resolution of inflammation.

Pain. As this is a chronic inflammatory process, pain is very rarely a feature of this disease. If pain is present it signifies the presence of some acute inflammatory condition such as Vincent's disease (acute ulcerative gingivitis), a periodontal abscess, acute herpetic gingivostomatitis or acute pericoronitis. Because pain is usually absent the disease may only be diagnosed at a very advanced stage, by which time it may be too late to save the teeth.

Mobility of the teeth. This is a very common symptom and is often the reason patients seek professional advice. Mobility may be localized to a single tooth or may be generalized, and results from loss of supporting tissues as a result of long-standing chronic periodontitis. Although chronic periodontitis is the most common cause of mobility of the teeth, other lesions such as neoplasms and

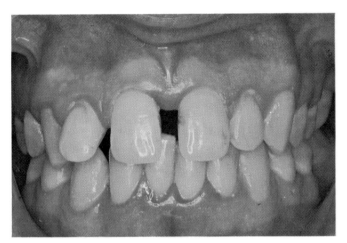

Figure 5.5. *Drifting and mobility of teeth affected by chronic periodontitis.*

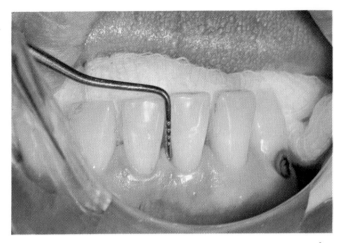

Figure 5.6. *The diagnosis and the measurement of a periodontal pocket.*

Figure 5.7. *Upper right quadrant illustrates an early chronic marginal gingivitis. Lower central incisors illustrate gingival disease of long duration.*

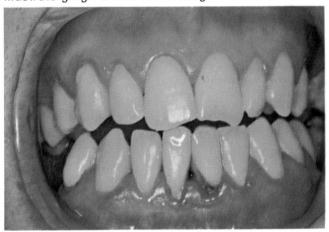

osteomyelitis could be responsible, and must be considered in a differential diagnosis.

The resolution of inflammation which follows the simple removal of calculus and plaque can reduce the mobility of teeth by as much as 25 per cent.

Drifting of the teeth. This again is a relatively common complication which results from an imbalance of forces as the consequence of loss of periodontal support. Spaces may appear in a dentition which was previously unaffected (Figure 5.5) and this could present a psychological problem to the patient because of an altered appearance of the anterior teeth. This complication can be corrected by restorative and orthodontic measures.

Halitosis and altered taste sensation. These are well-known complications of chronic periodontitis, and result from the accumulation and stagnation of food debris, blood and pus around the affected teeth.

Periodontal pockets. A periodontal pocket is defined as a pathologically deepened gingival crevice, and results from destruction of the fibres which anchor the tooth to the bone. This may or may not be accompanied by gingival recession, so that a diagnosis can only be made by careful probing of the gingival crevice. Pockets may vary in depth from 4 to 12 mm. The gingiva in chronic periodontitis may appear to be perfectly healthy to the untrained observer so that probing is sometimes the only way of making a definite diagnosis (Figure 5.6). If plaque accumulates in the depths of a pocket it is virtually impossible to remove by toothbrushing, and therefore it may be necessary to remove these pockets surgically. This allows access to plaque removal by the patient and dentist.

Figure 5.8. *Gross gingival hyperplasia as a result of long-standing inflammation.*

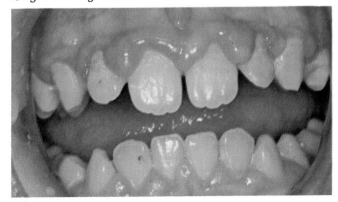

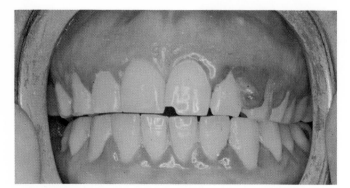

Figure 5.9. *Pregnancy epulis between upper left lateral incisor and canine tooth.*

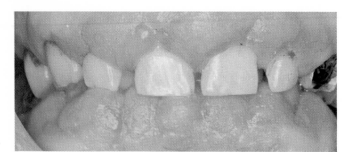

Figure 5.10. *Gingival enlargement following phenytoin administration.*

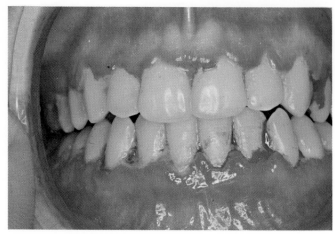

Figure 5.11. *Vincent's disease — trench mouth.*

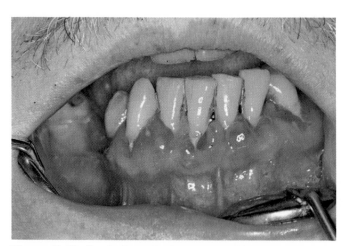

Figure 5.12. *Periodontal abscesses affecting the papillae of the lower anterior teeth.*

Figure 5.13. *Acute pericoronitis around lower left third molar.*

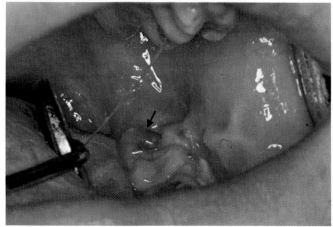

Inflammatory changes in the gingival margin. The very early signs of inflammation include redness of the gingival margin, loss of stippling due to oedema and distortion of the gingival margin which becomes rounded (Figure 5.7). Later the gum may become hyperplastic so that only part of the clinical crown is visible (Figure 5.8). This hyperplasia may be generalized or localized when it presents as a tumour-like growth known as an epulis. These consist of an excessive formation of granulation tissue very similar to the pyogenic granuloma seen in other parts of the body and are commonly associated with pregnancy (Figure 5.9). The swelling appears during the second trimester and can spontaneously regress following parturition. However, the tumour is unsightly, may bleed excessively and may have to be removed for these reasons. These lesions have a high tendency to recur, especially when associated with pregnancy. An increased severity of gingival inflammation has also been reported in women taking oral contraceptives. It is especially important therefore to ensure that patients who are pregnant or on the Pill practice a very high standard of plaque control.

Gingival enlargement can also follow the administration of drugs such as phenytoin (Figure 5.10) used in the treatment of epilepsy. The enlargement is due primarily to the effect of the drug on collagen synthesis so that the tissues may even be pink, stippled and firm. Treatment is surgical, but recurrence may follow unless the drug is withdrawn, which may not always be possible.

Acute Periodontitis

Although acute conditions of the periodontium are not as common as chronic periodontitis they can be very distressing to the patient and can present an alarming picture to the unwary practitioner. Treatment is simple and involves the use of drugs and surgery.

Acute Ulcerative Gingivitis (AUG, Vincent's Disease, Trench Mouth)

Acute ulcerative gingivitis is mainly a disease of adolescents or young adults. It affects the papillary portion of the gum which appears to be flattened, bleeds spontaneously and has a greyish slough over the ulcer which is the pathognomonic lesion (Figure 5.11). This is usually associated with a characteristic foetor oris (resulting from the presence of gangrenous tissue), regional lymphadenopathy and a pyrexia of 99 to 101°F.

The patient experiences intense pain, difficulty with eating, swallowing and even talking, and may complain of spontaneous haemorrhage or bleeding following eating.

Penicillin, metronidazole or nitrimidazine are considered to be the drugs of choice. Later treatment sometimes includes surgical correction of gingival deformities which may have resulted but certainly involves the complete removal of plaque and calculus.

Periodontal Abscess

This may be localized or generalized, single or multiple, and presents as a red, fluctuant swelling of the gingiva (Figure 5.12), which may be extremely tender to palpation. Abscesses are always associated with a periodontal pocket, with which they communicate, and pus can usually be expressed from the gingival crevice after probing. Treatment is surgical and is aimed at drainage of the pus. Periodontal abscesses are acute exacerbations of an existing chronic periodontitis.

Acute Pericoronitis

This term is usually reserved for acute inflammatory changes associated with gum flaps over partially erupted wisdom teeth (Figure 5.13). Inflammation may be localized or may spread to involve adjacent structures in the pharyngeal region, so that the patient may experience dysphagia or trismus. Treatment involves the administration of penicillin and the subsequent removal of the offending tooth.

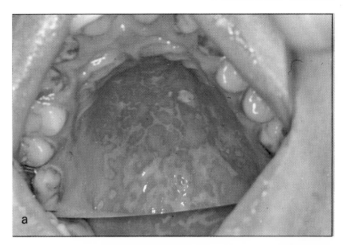

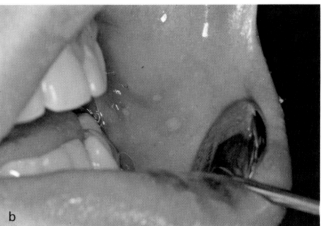

Figure 5.14. *(a) and (b) Acute herpetic gingivostomatitis in an adult.*

Acute Herpetic Gingivostomatitis

This condition commonly affects children between the ages of two and five years. It is characterized by a vesicular eruption of the oral mucosa which, because the vesicles burst rapidly, presents as small discrete shallow ulcers, or as large ulcers where these have coalesced (Figure 5.14). The patients will be extremely febrile and experience difficulty in eating and sleeping.

Clinically, the patient presents with marked regional lymphadenopathy, a temperature of 103 to 105°F, generalized ulceration of the mouth and lips, and redness and swelling of the gingiva.

This condition can be extremely worrying to the parents until they are made aware of the nature of the illness. The aetiology is viral, and treatment is palliative as the condition usually resolves in seven to ten days.

Intra-oral recurrence is extremely rare, but recurrent herpes labialis, usually confined to the lips and adjacent skin, is very common.

6. Orthodontic Disorders

Peter Vig

Orthodontics is the branch of dentistry concerned with the growth and development of the teeth and jaws. The orthodontist tries to treat positional anomalies of the teeth as they affect oral health and the physical, aesthetic and mental well-being of the patient.

The habit of regular dental attendance is often delayed or never acquired in childhood. In contrast, mothers are accustomed to taking their children to the family doctor shortly after birth. It is scarcely surprising that the family doctor is often in a better position than the dentist to notice problems of dento-facial development. Excluding such gross anomalies as clefts of the lips or palate (which occur in about 1 : 1,000 births) it has been estimated that from 30 to 60 per cent of children have a degree of irregularity of the teeth sufficient to be called a 'malocclusion'.

Malocclusion

Aetiology

In the past, crowding of the teeth, narrowness of the palatal vault and relative protrusion of either jaw were considered to be the result of disorders such as rickets, endocrine disturbance, mouth breathing due to the occlusion of the nasal airway—especially by adenoids—and inadequate function which failed to stimulate growth. These ideas have been disproved and replaced by a more biological approach to the aetiology and the treatment of malocclusion.

The development of dental occlusion is now known to be a result of three major factors. These are first, the dental features such as size, shape, number and develop-

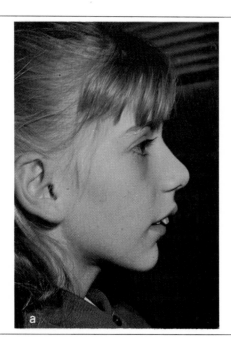

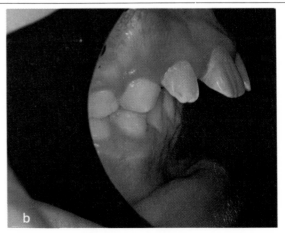

Figure 6.1. *(a) Despite lips-apart posture, this girl is not a mouth breather. Nasal respiration is maintained by the formation of a posterior oral seal between the dorsum of the tongue and the soft palate. (b) Incisor relationship — upper incisors proclined.*

mental position of the teeth (Figure 6.1). Second, the relationship between the maxilla and mandible which determines the spatial relationship of the opposing dental arches (Figure 6.2). Third, the effect over a period of time of forces exerted by the tongue, lips and cheeks.

The response to physiological forces acting on teeth is tooth migration through the supporting alveolar bone. This fact is not only responsible for the ultimate position of the teeth, but is also why orthodontic treatment by tooth movement is possible.

All these factors, i.e. dental, skeletal and neuromuscular patterns, are genetically determined. The mode of inheritance of each group of features is independent and subject to a wide range of normal variation. It is thus evident that the development of dental and facial relationships is predicated on multifactorial genetic variations, and it is therefore to be expected that throughout the population there exists an infinite range of variation in dental and facial arrangement.

Should the inherited features in the individual combine to make up a harmonious whole, the resulting clinical picture is acceptable or normal. If, however, there is sufficient disharmony between the parts, an unacceptable dental or facial configuration develops. The cases which form the larger proportion of orthodontic problems are therefore not abnormal individuals, but simply normal variations which deviate from an arbitrary norm for the community.

Timing of Treatment

Although malocclusion may be evident in the primary or early mixed dentition, with a few exceptions, orthodontic treatment is best delayed until the shedding of the primary teeth has taken place, and the permanent canines and premolars have erupted (Figure 6.3). For most children this is from 11 to 13 years. Since this may mean a delay of several years after the recognition of the condition, it is often necessary to reassure the anxious parent that it is to the child's advantage that no immediate action be taken. There are reasons for this delay. It is not possible to influence the position of the permanent successors by orthodontic movement of the primary teeth. It is therefore necessary to allow the permanent teeth to erupt irrespective of their position. The nature and severity of a malocclusion are determined by growth and development of the cranio-facial skeleton and oropharyngeal musculature. Maturation of the various structures occurs at differing rates. Although most of the growth potential of the facial skeleton has been realized by the early teens, the mandible can continue to grow until the early twenties. Differential development of the tooth-bearing bones will, of course, influence the relationship between the upper and lower dental arches.

Prediction of amount and direction of growth is one of the orthodontist's problems. Growth not only determines the natural course of dental development but will also determine the prognosis of orthodontic treatment in terms of the stability of the result.

The overall type of skeletal pattern becomes evident in the first year of life. But prediction with any degree of precision is difficult until after the growth spurt which occurs at puberty. This is another factor which may influence the orthodontist in the timing of his treatment.

Certain irregularities of dental development, however,

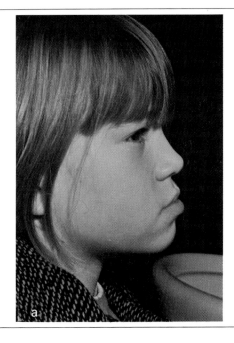
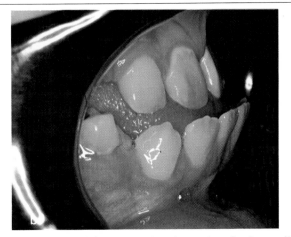

Figure 6.2. *(a) This patient's malocclusion will worsen as she grows older. (b) As the mandible continues its downward and forward growth, the lower incisors will be carried further away from the upper incisors.*

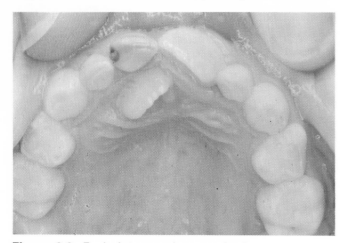

Figure 6.3. *Early intervention required.*

Figure 6.4. *A common complaint. The displaced maxillary incisor requires early treatment.*

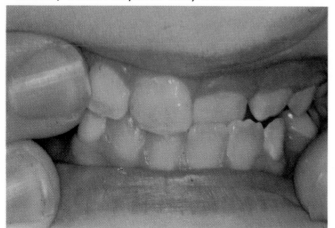

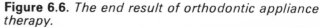

Figure 6.5. *A malocclusion.*

Figure 6.6. *The end result of orthodontic appliance therapy.*

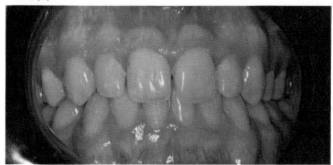

should be treated early (i.e. in the mixed primary dentition). Perhaps the most common of these conditions is the eruption of an upper permanent incisor such that it occludes behind the lower incisors (Figure 6.4). This reversed incisor relationship usually affects one tooth, but may in some cases affect all four upper incisors (Figure 6.5). Where a central incisor tooth is involved, it becomes apparent by about the eighth year. A few months of appliance therapy, with or without the extraction of some primary teeth to produce adequate space, can correct this situation (Figure 6.6).

Occasionally by about eight years it becomes apparent that an upper central incisor has failed to erupt. This should be investigated without delay. The congenital absence of upper central incisors is extremely rare (the wisdom teeth, second premolars and upper lateral incisors are the teeth most frequently missing). Any delay in eruption, which may be due to a number of causes, should be diagnosed, and the appropriate treatment commenced.

Eruption of lower permanent incisors before the shedding of their primary precursors is quite common. The wider crowns of the permanent teeth lead to crowding with displacement and rotation of these teeth. This condition is seen in seven-year-olds (Figure 6.7). Parents are usually worried by what they call 'double teeth'. No treatment is required at this stage. Spontaneous alignment often results after the shedding of all the primary teeth. If crowding persists, this will have to be treated in the permanent dentition.

Normally, when closing from rest to a tooth together position, the mandible moves in an upward and forward arc. If, however, the position of one or more teeth interferes with this normally symmetrical movement, a 'mandibular displacement' may occur. The altered path of closure is reflexly established and maintained and is initiated by an uncomfortable or traumatic occlusion (see Figure 6.8).

The removal of the cause of this abnormal pattern of

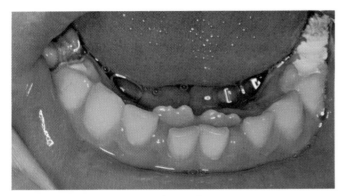

Figure 6.7. *Normal eruption of lower incisors, not a malocclusion.*

Figure 6.8. *This may or may not be immediately treated — this patient requires an early orthodontic assessment.*

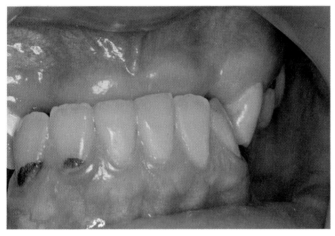

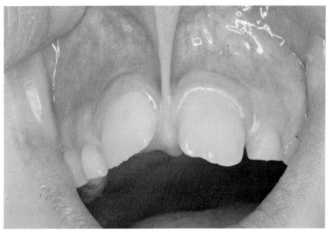

Figure 6.9. *No immediate intervention is necessary for the young patient's lower labial fraenum.*

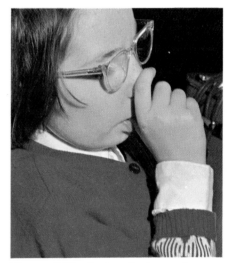

Figure 6.10. *A classical pose!*

mandibular movement is indicated. The first symptoms of such a condition may be pain, clicking or limitation of movement in one or both temporomandibular joints. Since patients do not appreciate the dental nature of their problem, many such patients first see their medical practitioner.

Some Occasions when Treatment is not Needed

Having pointed out the limitations of orthodontic treatment in the primary dentition, reassurance from the doctor may also help in a number of other cases not requiring immediate treatment.

Mothers are often concerned at the unsightly gap which may exist between the upper permanent central incisors shortly after they erupt. Frequently, this space appears to be associated with the insertion of the labial fraenum (Figure 6.9). In most cases fraenectomy and orthodontic treatment are unnecessary. The majority of such spaces

Figure 6.11. *Anterior open bite.*

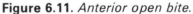

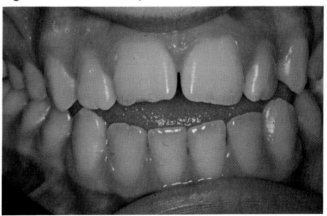

7. Attrition, Abrasion, Erosion and the Temporomandibular Joint

C. E. Renson

This chapter is concerned with conditions related to tooth tissue loss not usually associated with the commonest cause of such loss, viz. dental caries.

By their very nature attrition, abrasion, erosion and temporomandibular joint (TMJ) symptoms are found in adults, rather than in children, and frequently affect more elderly patients. There are, however, exceptions to this rule and they will be dealt with in the course of this chapter.

In the elderly patient who presents with a number of remaining natural teeth, which look as if they are worn down almost to gum level, it is probable that the three conditions have been or are present, although it is often difficult to separate them as entities (Figure 7.1). For ease of description, however, they are best dealt with separately.

Attrition

Attrition is the process of wearing away of tooth surfaces as a result of grinding opposing teeth. This may be associated with mastication or grinding the teeth at night (bruxism), or as an unconscious habit during the day. The diet of Western civilized man is such that mastication alone is unlikely to lead to gross wear, even during a lifetime. The same cannot be said of some primitive peoples, e.g. the aborigines of Australia, or of some items of 'diet' which are constantly chewed, e.g. tobacco which contains sand particles (Figure 7.2), and betel-nuts (Figure 7.3) (a favourite with many Asian peoples), which are sprinkled with ground sea shells or coral. In modern Western man the most significant cause of attrition is bruxism (Figure 7.4) and this is frequently associated with an underlying anxiety.

Another important predisposing factor of attrition is hypoplasia of the teeth (see page 6) and when this is general throughout the mouth, it may lead to considerable wear.

Attrition may also affect the contact areas, i.e. the approximal surfaces of the teeth and is caused by friction

Figure 7.1. *A male patient, 65 years of age, who presented with his remaining maxillary teeth severely attrited, abraded and eroded and an early history of persistent regurgitation of food 20 years earlier.*

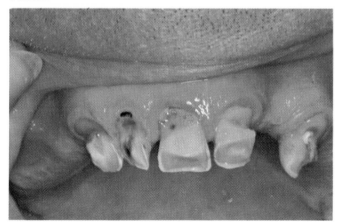

Figure 7.2. *The maxillary teeth of a habitual tobacco chewer, a merchant seaman. More wear is usually seen in the palatal cusps of upper teeth and the buccal cusps of lower teeth. The exposed dentine is stained.*

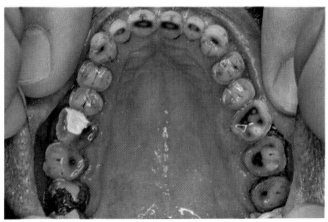

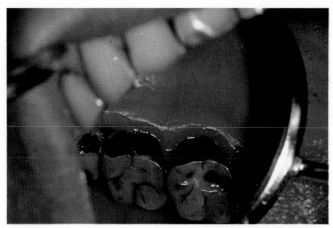

Figure 7.3. *Marked abrasion of the maxillary molars in a betel-nut chewer. The betel-nut is the fruit of the areca palm and is commonly chewed by many people in India, Ceylon, Malaysia and other Asian countries. Tooth wear is accelerated by the addition of powdered coral or ground sea shells to the betel-nut; a not uncommon practice in these countries.*

Figure 7.4. *Tooth wear caused by bruxism in a white male, 40 years of age. Bruxism is the habit of grinding the teeth when asleep and this may continue during the day. It is accepted that this is a response to tension and anxiety. Where teeth do not occlude correctly the mandible has to twist and the temporomandibular joint is similarly twisted.*

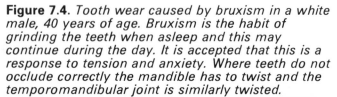

Figure 7.5. *Early attrition in a female patient, 43 years of age. Only part of the enamel has been removed from the incisal and occlusal surfaces of the maxillary teeth.*

Figure 7.6. *Gross attrition in a male, 50 years of age. The whole of the grinding enamel has been worn away and because the underlying dentine is softer it wears much more rapidly than the enamel left at the margins.*

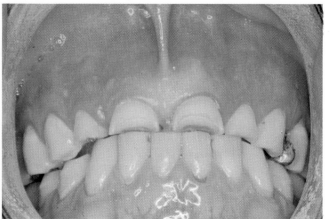

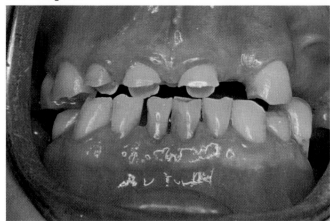

brought about by grinding. In the early stages of attrition only part of the enamel is removed from incisal and occlusal surfaces (Figure 7.5) but over a period the whole of the grinding enamel may disappear, uncovering the underlying dentine. Dentine wears much more rapidly than the enamel left at the margins and shallow concavities form in the dentine surrounded by enamel which is 'proud' of the dentine (Figure 7.6). The pulp of the tooth is protected by the formation of secondary dentine (see page 22). Pain is rarely associated with such wear until pulpal exposure occurs at a very late date (Figure 7.7) or until overclosure of the mandible consequent upon the wear positions the head of the condyle in the glenoid fossa in such a way as to lead to temporomandibular joint malfunction.

Treatment

If the cause is tobacco or betel-nut chewing, this should be discouraged. If the cause is bruxism, and often the

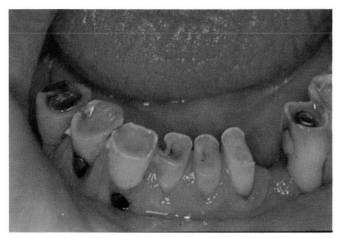

Figure 7.7. *Gross attrition in a male, 65 years of age. The pulps of the teeth have remained protected by the production of reparative dentine until this very late stage when pulpal exposure of the lower incisors has occurred.*

Figure 7.8. *A clear acrylic splint is often prescribed where attrition caused by bruxism has caused related joint pain or dysfunction. The splint is worn at night, and in some cases during the day. It halts the wear process, serves to equilibrate the occlusion and discourages the habit of grinding the teeth.*

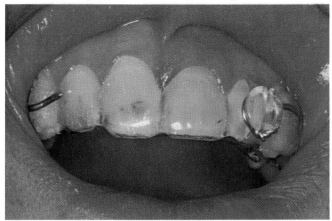

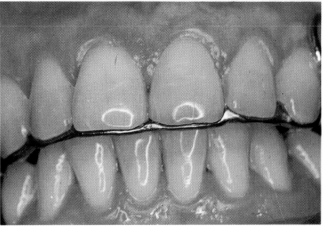

Figure 7.9. *In some cases metal overlays have to be prescribed as a permanency to equilibrate the occlusion and thus overcome further deterioration of the TMJ condition and to prevent additional wear of the teeth. This may be in the form of a metal removable dental splint (as shown here) or in the form of metal fillings permanently inserted into the teeth, whichever is thought more appropriate.*

patient's spouse will be aware of the habit and the patient unaware, then referral to a dental surgeon is indicated. The dentist may place a transparent plastic occlusal splint (Figure 7.8) which will halt the wear process and may serve to discourage the habit. The splint is frequently helpful if TMJ pain and/or clicking is present, and in this connection there are exercises which the patient can perform to relax the spasm of the external pterygoid muscle, frequently associated with TMJ trouble. The plastic splint may be followed by a metal overlay on the worn surfaces in the form of separate gold fillings or a metal splint (Figure 7.9).

Frost (1972) described a sign which is pathognomonic of pain of TMJ origin. He calls it the 'pterygoid sign' and elicits it in the following manner:

'The examiner faces the patient and, to examine the right side, places the tip of the little finger of his right hand above and slightly behind the maxillary tuberosity. If the patient winces the sign is positive. If the patient does not wince the sign is negative. To examine the left side the tip of the left little finger is used.'

In several thousand cases Frost claims only two possible false negatives. If palpation is gently done, false positives do not occur. If the sign is present, TMJ disease is present though not necessarily the cause of the pain complained of. If the sign is absent the pain complained of is not of TMJ origin. Temporomandibular joint symptoms are frequently psychosomatic in origin and in these cases Frost's sign may prove invaluable.

A clinical observation of the author has been that young women who present with TMJ symptoms will sometimes reveal, after careful questioning, that the current male consort is somewhat vigorous in his osculatory activities—a gentle word of advice frequently seems to resolve the condition in these circumstances! Attrition and

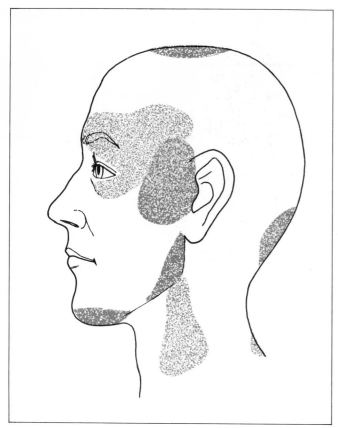

Figure 7.10. *Distribution of facial and head pain arising from temporomandibular joint dysfunction.*

Figure 7.11. *Toothbrush abrasion shown as 'V'-shaped notches at the necks of the mandibular canine and first premolar (the other teeth are on a partial denture). This is brought about by the incorrect use of the toothbrush and occurs in this situation because gum recession has uncovered the enamel–cementum junction.*

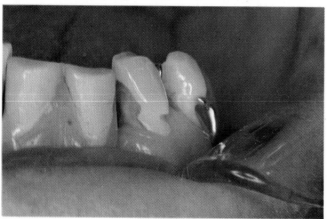

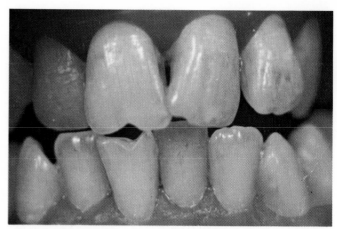

Figure 7.12. *The notches in the incisal edges of the upper central incisor and the opposing lower central incisor were produced by the repeated use of these teeth to open hair-clips.*

bruxism are not, of course, the only causes of temporomandibular joint disease or malfunction. In TMJ pain (Figure 7.10) and clicking which persists after the restoration of correct occlusal height, the replacement of missing teeth, the elimination of early contact on closing and exercises to relax muscle spasm, the following conditions must be remembered: rheumatoid arthritis, osteoarthritis and arthrosis. In these conditions short-wave therapy may be helpful. Some workers have found that the injection of a saline suspension of hydrocortisone acetate or local anaesthetics into the joint has achieved some success. As a last resort excision of the condyle may be carried out, but this should be a rare necessity.

Abrasion

Abrasion of tooth tissue is caused by the friction of a foreign body or substance. The commonest form of abrasion is associated with the incorrect use of the toothbrush. Using a toothbrush with a sawing-like motion will produce a series of V-shaped notches at the necks of teeth (Figure 7.11); in right-handed people the teeth on the left side are most affected and vice versa. This type of defect is seen most frequently where some gum recession has occurred uncovering the less abrasion-resistant tissue at the enamel–cementum junction of the tooth. If enamel is involved it is by being undermined, because the toothbrush bristles and most modern toothpastes are insufficiently abrasive to cause wear of enamel. The misuse of dental floss and tooth picks may also lead to this type of abrasion. Pipe-smoking may lead to the abrasion of anterior teeth. Certain occupations can also be associated with tooth abrasion, e.g. the seamstress who constantly

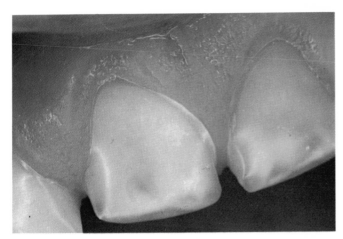

Figure 7.13. *Erosion of the upper anterior teeth in a patient who repeatedly regurgitated his food over a lengthy period.*

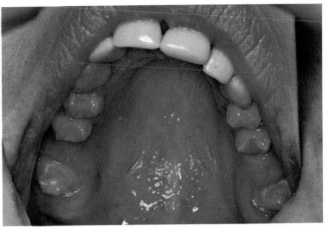

Figure 7.14. *Erosion of the teeth in a woman, 36 years of age, who had persistently taken hot pure lemon juice each night for two years on retiring, in the belief that it would induce weight reduction. All the teeth in both jaws were affected, but the anterior teeth in the illustration have been crowned by her dentist.*

'bites off' the thread, the hairdresser who holds hair-clips between her teeth (Figure 7.12). Treatment usually consists of correcting the faulty habit and placing fillings where these are necessary.

Erosion

Erosion of teeth is generally regarded as being caused by an acid disintegration of tooth tissue not associated with bacteria. The repeated regurgitation of food from the stomach has been reported as a cause (Figure 7.13), and the taking of dilute hydrochloric acid in patients suffering from hypochlorhydria. Workers in chemical plants where acids are used have tooth erosion, particularly on the anterior teeth which are least protected by the soft tissues from the fumes. Citric acid in all its forms is highly destructive of tooth tissue and people who habitually suck lemons, oranges or grapefruit may exhibit erosion. The drinking of lemon juice as 'an aid to slimming' can also have quite disastrous dental effects (Figure 7.14). There can be little doubt that the free orange juice made available for many years in Britain was responsible for much destruction of tooth tissue in young mothers. The anterior 'ring' of missing tooth tissue in very young children was frequently caused by the continuous sucking of sweetened orange juice from bottles (see page 22).

There are patients who present with tooth erosion in which no convincing history can be obtained related to the presence of acid. This is idiopathic erosion. The lesions are saucer-shaped and they originate in enamel rather than

Figure 7.15. *Idiopathic erosion cavities in the upper central incisor teeth of a woman, 35 years of age. Characteristically the lesions are saucer-shaped and originate in enamel and not dentine or cementum, as do other types of erosion.*

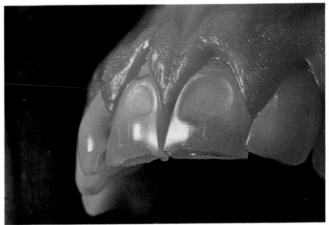

on the root surface. Incisors and premolars are most frequently affected. The surface is hard which differentiates it from caries (Figure 7.15). Treatment of erosion consists of fillings for the lesions and appropriate advice where acid is incriminated.

Reference
Frost, M., *Br. Dent. J.*, 1972, **132**, 51.

Section 3
Diseases of the Oral Mucosa and Jaws

8. Ulcers of the Oral Mucosa

J. Lozdan

Lesions of the oral mucosa may present originally as macules, papules, nodules, tumours, plaques, vesicles, bullae, pustules, erosions and ulcers. The most common of these clinical forms is the ulcer. Any lesion, irrespective of its original morphology, may become modified to present as an ulcer. This is because the oral mucosa is constantly subjected to the potentially damaging actions of chewing and swallowing hot and cold, rough and hard particles of food and to various chemicals contained in food or dissolved in the saliva. The clinical presentation and progress of ulcers will also be affected by oral debris, saliva and the many organisms which constitute the commensal flora of the mouth.

It seems remarkable that the oral mucosa manages to maintain its integrity so successfully in these circumstances and does not ulcerate more frequently. This integrity of the oral mucosa is maintained by a balance between the resistance of the tissues and damaging external and internal influences. Whenever there is an imbalance between these factors, an ulcer may result. Thus in leukaemia (Figure 8.1) or agranulocytosis, the ability of tissues to repair in the presence of traumatic or infective influences is severely impaired and an ulcer may occur. The pathogenesis of any ulcer of the oral mucosa while dominated by a single aetiological factor, may be affected by a wide variety of influences. The investigation and treatment of oral ulcers must therefore take into account focal and systemic factors.

Oral ulcers may present the general practitioner with difficult diagnostic and therapeutic problems. This is because, although their aetiology may be diverse, clinically the lesions may have similar appearances. In many cases the aetiology is speculative, if not unknown, so that the treatment is only palliative and not curative. This has prompted the production of a spate of products which may be used for the treatment of these lesions. It is a mistake, however, to encourage self-treatment, as many potentially dangerous ulcers may go unrecognized.

Most ulcers are painful and may interfere with chewing, swallowing, nutrition and even speech.

For descriptive purposes oral ulcers may be divided into the following types:

1. Those in which the ulcers are confined to the oral mucosa.

2. Those in which similar lesions are found on the skin or other mucous membranes.

3. Those associated with general systemic disease.

Ulcers Confined to the Mouth

Recurrent Aphthous Ulceration

Canker sores, dyspeptic aphthosis, vesicular stomatitis and ulcerative stomatitis. This entity is by far the commonest form of oral ulceration. The aetiology is unknown but many interesting hypotheses have been advanced. Emotional factors, allergy, viral or bacterial influences, hormonal imbalance, trauma, anaemia, nutritional deficiencies, gastrointestinal disturbances and auto-immune reactions have all been incriminated.

Clinically these ulcers may be subdivided into three categories:

1. Minor aphthous ulcers (MiAU)

2. Major aphthous ulcers (MjAU)

3. Herpetiform ulcers

Minor aphthous ulceration. These ulcers affect women more than men—they may occur at any age but are more frequently seen between 10 and 20 years of age. They may involve any area of the oral mucosa but are normally confined to the lips and cheeks.

Typically the patient will give a history of an initial burning or itching sensation of the oral mucosa which is followed by the appearance of one to four shallow oral ulcers, 3 to 10 mm in diameter and surrounded by an area of erythema (Figure 8.2). The ulcers are exquisitely painful but usually heal within seven to ten days without scarring.

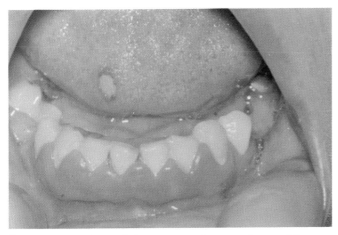

Figure 8.1. *Ulcer of the tongue in a patient with leukaemia.*

Figure 8.2. *Recurrent aphthae affecting the palate and fauces.*

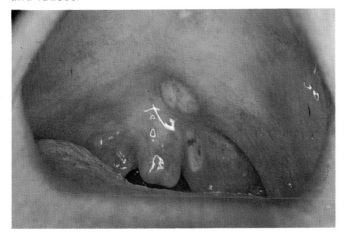

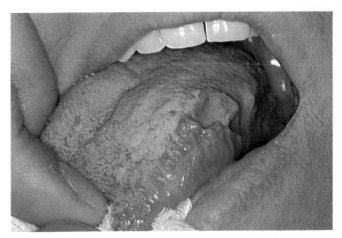

Figure 8.3. *Major aphthous ulceration of side of tongue.*

Figure 8.4. *Herpetiform ulceration of the palate.*

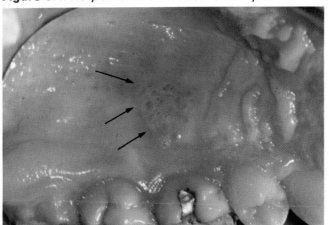

Major aphthous ulceration. Major aphthous ulcers are considered to be a more severe form of the minor variety. In addition to the lips and cheeks, these lesions may also be seen on the tongue, soft palate and pharynx. The ulcers are much larger (more than 10 mm in diameter) and deeper than the minor variety and may be accompanied by regional lymphadenopathy (Figure 8.3). They take up to six weeks to heal and often result in scarring. In a small percentage of cases scarring may be very severe, sufficient to cause deformities of the lips and tongue.

Herpetiform ulcers. These are described as herpetiform because they resemble in size and shape the ulcers seen in acute herpetic gingivostomatitis. However, a viral aetiology has not been established. The patient may present with crops of 5 to 100 shallow ulcers most of which are between 2 to 5 mm in diameter (Figure 8.4). Occasionally a crop of ulcers may coalesce so that a single ulcer more then 10 mm in diameter may be seen. The ulcers heal without scarring within seven to ten days.

All aphthous ulcers may precede or be part of Behcet's or Reiter's syndrome, which will be discussed later.

As the aetiology is unknown the treatment of these ulcers can only be palliative and empirical. Local steroid therapy in the form of either hydrocortisone–succinate or beta-methasone-17-valerate pellets or in a gel combined with an adhesive vehicle (Adcortyl A—in Orabase R), have been used for the treatment of MiAU and MjAU, while herpetiform ulcers appear to respond better to a two per cent suspension of tetracycline as a mouthwash. Rarely, severe episodes of major aphthous ulceration warrant the use of systemic steroids.

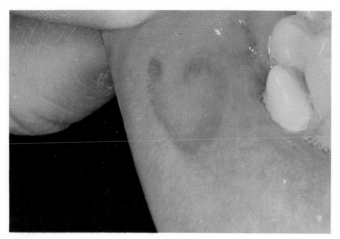

Figure 8.5. *Traumatic ulcer following lip biting.*

Figure 8.6. *(a) Ulcers of the lip mucosa in a patient with herpes zoster. (b) Unilateral mouth and skin lesions in patient with herpes zoster.*

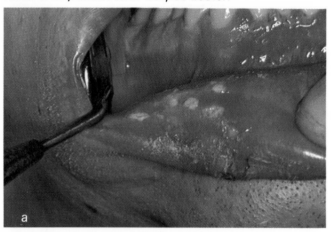

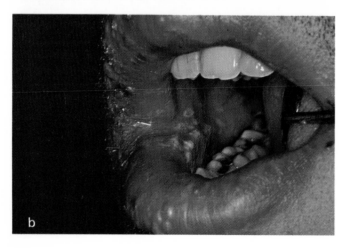

Traumatic Ulcers

Apart from the local factors already mentioned, the oral mucosa may be traumatized by dentures and other prosthetic appliances, the jagged margins of restorations and decayed teeth and the over-zealous use of a tooth-brush. Occasionally a traumatic ulcer may follow biting of the lip or cheek (Figure 8.5). This may follow dental treatment when the patient may be unaware that he is damaging anaesthetized tissues. Traumatic ulcers are characterized by irregular and ragged margins and vary in size and shape. A careful history and examination of the mouth will often reveal the traumatic influence.

Treatment is directed at removal of the cause which will be followed by healing within seven to ten days. During the healing phase the ulcer can be protected by a surface covering of Orabase.

All traumatic ulcers which have not healed within two weeks of the identification and removal of the cause should be biopsied to eliminate the possibility of malignancy.

Acute Herpetic Gingivostomatitis

The oral mucosa is affected in the primary attack of the herpes simplex virus. This condition occurs most commonly in children between two and five years of age, although it can be seen in adults (see page 50). The initial symptoms are those of a sore throat, enlarged submandibular lymph nodes, and a burning sensation of the oral mucosa. This is soon followed by a vesicular eruption of the mucosa which, unlike that on the skin, soon ruptures to produce ulcers. These may be small at first but they often coalesce into large shallow ulcers with serpiginous borders. All areas of the mouth may be affected and there is usually a generalized enlargement and redness of the gingival mucosa. The patient is febrile and has difficulty with talking, eating and swallowing. The condition normally resolves within seven to ten days. Treatment is palliative and involves a high fluid intake, a semifluid diet, the administration of a soothing mouthwash (glycerine and thymol) and the use of antibiotics to control secondary infection. Patients must be warned not to touch their eyes as this may result in herpetic corneal ulceration.

Diagnosis can be confirmed by the harvesting of cells from the periphery of the ulcer within the first five days. The virus can be isolated by culture or the typical intra-nuclear inclusion bodies can be found microscopically. It should also be possible to demonstrate a rising titre of antibodies during the convalescence period. Recurrence in the oral mucosa is extremely rare but recurrent herpes labialis, usually confined to the lips and adjacent skin, is very common.

Herpes Zoster

Patients with herpes zoster will always give a history of having had varicella, as the same virus is responsible for both conditions. The pathology and clinical appearances of the oral mucosal lesions are similar to those of acute herpetic gingivostomatitis. However, in herpes zoster the lesions are usually unilateral and involve dermatomes associated with branches of the trigeminal nerve (Figure 8.6). In some cases severe complications such as corneal ulceration, postherpetic neuralgia and facial palsy may follow an infection with this virus. Treatment involves the use of antibiotics to control secondary infection.

Herpangina and Hand–foot and Mouth Disease

Both of these diseases are caused by infection from the coxsackie group of viruses. Herpangina principally affects children and is characterized by the appearance of multiple small ulcers mainly on the soft palate and pharynx. The onset is sudden and the patient presents with a fever, a sore throat and regional lymphadenopathy. The disease is self-limiting and usually resolves within a week. Hand–foot and mouth disease is characterized by the presence of oral ulcers associated with skin lesions of the hands and feet. Oral lesions are clinically indistinguishable from minor aphthous ulceration. The disease usually resolves within 10 days.

Candidiasis

Acute and chronic candidiasis of the oral mucosa can produce severe ulceration. Acute candidiasis usually affects infants but may also be seen in adults following the administration of antibiotics which upset the balance of the bacterial flora in the mouth, and in patients who are severely debilitated, suffering from diabetes and on corticosteroid or cytotoxic therapy. Acute candidiasis presents as white milk curd patches on the oral mucosa which at first can be wiped off to reveal a bleeding ulcerated surface (Figure 8.7). Chronic atrophic candidiasis (also known as denture stomatitis) is usually associated with the wearing of dentures and presents as an erythematous, eroded area of the oral mucosa associated with the fitting surface of the upper denture (Figure 8.8). This condition may or may not be accompanied by angular cheilosis (Figure 8.9). Predisposing factors may be anaemia, pregnancy, diabetes or steroid therapy.

Diagnosis is confirmed by taking smears either from the mucosa or the surface of the denture. These will reveal the typical hyphal and yeast forms of *Candida albicans*. Local therapy involves the treatment of the predisposing cause and the administration of either nystatin (500,000 i.u.) or amphotericin B lozenges (10 mg), which are sucked four

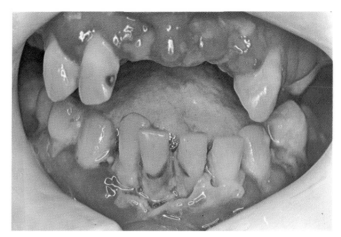

Figure 8.7. *Acute candidiasis.*

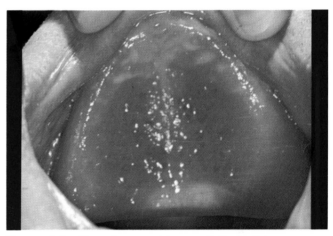

Figure 8.8. *Chronic atrophic candidiasis ('denture stomatitis').*

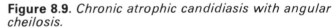

Figure 8.9. *Chronic atrophic candidiasis with angular cheilosis.*

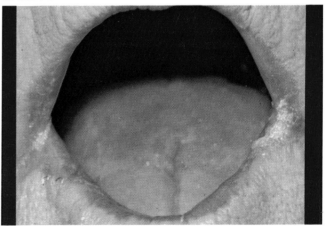

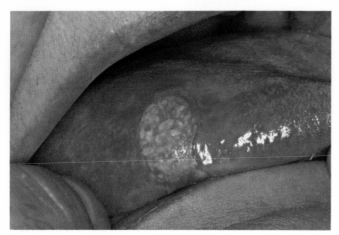

Figure 8.10. *Carcinoma of the tongue.*

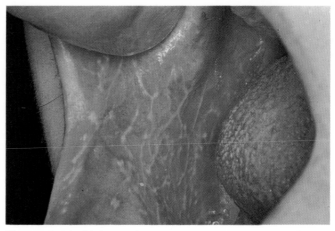

Figure 8.11. *Lichen planus.*

times a day often for one month. Attention should be paid to denture hygiene and new dentures may be required.

Syphilis and Tuberculosis

These conditions may present as chronic ulcers of the oral mucosa. Diagnosis is made from the typical history of these conditions and the demonstration of specific organisms. Syphilis is considered in more detail in Chapter 9.

Carcinoma of the Mouth

Any ulcer of the mouth which has persisted for more than two weeks should be regarded with suspicion and a biopsy performed. A malignant ulcer will present with induration of the base and limitation of movement of the affected part. The most common sites are the lip and lateral margins of the tongue (Figure 8.10). It is important therefore in any examination of the mouth to pull the tongue well forward to examine the lateral margins carefully. This easy visibility and accessibility to lesions in the mouth should allow an early diagnosis of carcinoma to be made. Early diagnosis and treatment are imperative if a cure is to be established. A suspicious lesion therefore should be regarded as an urgent diagnostic problem. Treatment involves radiotherapy or surgery.

Oral Ulcers Associated with Similar Lesions of the Skin and Other Mucous Membranes

All of the following diseases may present with oral lesions, either alone or as part of a general mucocutaneous eruption. When the skin is involved, patients are best treated in collaboration with a dermatologist. Oral lesions may precede the cutaneous eruption by months or even years. Occasionally, however, oral lesions may persist after the skin lesions have disappeared and these may present the clinician with difficult therapeutic problems for which there is no easy answer. Those diseases which characteristically present as vesicular or bullous eruptions of the skin have a different form in the mouth, for bullae are usually shortlived, breaking down to produce ulcers. Diagnosis depends primarily on the clinical examination as the histological findings in mucosal biopsies (except for pemphigus) are fairly non-specific. When teeth are present, the condition known as desquamative gingivitis may be an accompaniment of these diseases.

Extraction of the teeth may afford only temporary relief as new lesions can be associated or precipitated by the wearing of dentures. Most of these diseases are treated by the local administration of steroids when the mouth only is affected or by systemic steroids when associated with skin lesions.

Lichen Planus

Lichen planus may present in the mouth as a white patch, an erythematous atrophic area, or as an ulcer. A white pattern (resembling fine lacework), composed of multiple confluent papules may be seen (Figure 8.11). Lesions are usually bilaterally symmetrical. Lichen planus may affect the oral mucosa alone or the skin may also be involved. Oral lesions, like those on the skin, appear to be associated or precipitated by trauma and this may be the reason that they are more commonly seen on the cheeks and the tongue. When the teeth are present the condition known as desquamative gingivitis may be seen. The gingivae are fiery red, glazed and they present with varying degrees of erosion, ulceration and even vesiculation (Figure 8.12).

Treatment involves the administration of betamethasone-17-valerate 0.1 mg tablets, four to six of which are sucked daily. This treatment is often helpful although

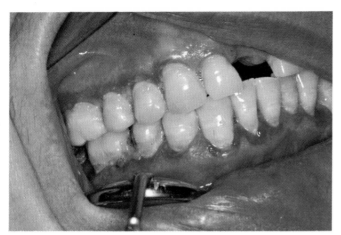

Figure 8.12. *Desquamative gingivitis associated with lichen planus.*

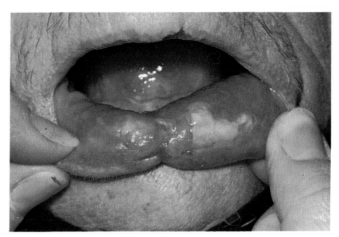

Figure 8.13. *Pemphigus vulgaris.*

lesions may recur and persist for years. Occasionally there are spontaneous remissions. If local steroid therapy does not control the lesions systemic therapy may be indicated.

Pemphigus

The oral lesions of pemphigus vulgaris and vegetans may be the first manifestations of the disease. The onset is usually between 30 and 50 years of age. Both sexes are equally affected. Patients present with large ulcers of the mucosa which have a thin white cuff at the periphery, representing the remnants of the burst bullae. All parts of the oral mucosa may be affected, but the common sites are the non-keratinized areas such as the cheeks, lips (Figure 8.13), floor of the mouth and ventral surface of the tongue. Nikolsky's test, elicited by either rubbing the mucosa or by a blast of air, is positive if this mild trauma produces a typical bulla. Smears taken either from the periphery of ulcers or from an intact bulla show the typical acantholytic or Tzanck cells.

Oral lesions may be controlled by local steroid therapy. Systemic steroid therapy is indicated in resistant cases and those associated with skin lesions and systemic effects.

Pemphigoid (Benign Mucous Membrane Pemphigus or Pemphigoid, Cicatricial Pemphigoid)

This disease is usually found in elderly women over 50 years of age. It can affect the mucous membranes of the mouth, nose, pharynx, larynx, oesophagus, skin and the eye. Ocular lesions may be particularly serious and can lead to scarring and even blindness. This complication may be prevented if an early diagnosis can be established by the recognition of lesions when they affect oral mucosa alone. The characteristic appearance in the oral mucosa is

that of large ulcers surrounded by tags of epithelium. Occasionally an intact bulla may be observed but this is unusual (Figure 8.14). Unlike pemphigus the disease affects the keratinized parts of the oral mucosa such as that covering the palate (Figure 8.15), dorsum of the tongue and the alveolar ridges. As in lichen planus when teeth are present, desquamative gingivitis is seen in addition to bullae and ulcers.

Lesions often heal with scarring, and adhesions may result where two mucosal surfaces are in close contact. When other mucosal surfaces are affected, patients may complain of nose bleeds, hoarseness of the throat and difficulty in swallowing. Treatment often may involve close liaison with ophthalmologists, dermatologists and otolaryngologists. The main condition from which pemphigoid has to be differentiated is pemphigus. Although Nikolsky's sign may be present in both, pemphigoid is characterized by a long history, the absence of acantholytic cells on smears and the histological demonstration of sub-epithelial vesicles. Lesions are usually well controlled by the use of local steroid therapy.

Erythema Multiforme (Stevens–Johnson Syndrome)

This disease can affect the mouth alone or may occur in conjunction with ocular, genital and skin lesions in which case it is referred to as Stevens–Johnson syndrome. The aetiology is unknown but may follow the use of drugs such as sulphonamides, penicillin and barbiturates. Occasionally, erythema multiforme may be preceded by a bout of recurrent herpetic infection affecting the lips. Several cases have been associated with infection by mycoplasma pneumonia. The onset of the condition is sudden and the whole attack usually lasts from two to three weeks. Patients are usually febrile, have enlarged cervical lymph nodes, a temperature of 101°F and experience great dis-

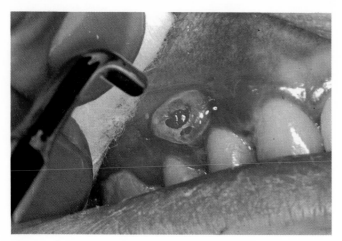

Figure 8.14. *An intact pemphigoid bulla.*

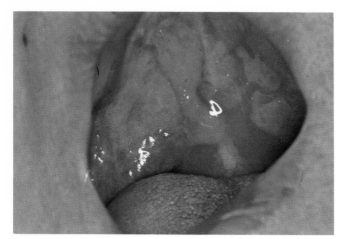

Figure 8.15. *Pemphigoid of the palatal mucosa.*

Figure 8.16. *Erythema multiforme.*

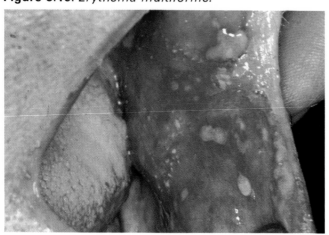

comfort when talking, chewing and swallowing.

The oral mucosa presents with large, erythematous, shallow ulcers covered with haemorrhagic fibrinous sloughs (Figure 8.16). Almost the whole of the oral mucosa with the exception of the gingivae may be involved. On the skin an extensive erythematous or macular rash may be present, associated with the classical 'iris' or 'target'-like lesions on the palms of the hands and soles of the feet. The infective component of the oral lesions alone is initially controlled by the administration of tetracycline 250 mg q.d.s. for seven days. This may be followed by local steroid therapy.

Behcet's Syndrome

Behcet's syndrome is classically described as consisting of a triple symptom complex of anterior uveitis with oral and genital ulceration. In recent years other features have been added. These include erythema nodosum, erythema multiforme and pyoderma, neurological involvement in 20 per cent of cases, and non-suppurative arthritis in 30 per cent of cases. In the mouth, intermittent oral ulceration indistinguishable from aphthae of either the major or minor variety may be seen. The oral ulcers are best treated by the local application of steroids.

Oral Ulceration Associated with General Systemic Disease

Oral ulceration may be a complication of many systemic diseases. Haematological disorders usually associated with oral ulceration include acute leukaemia, agranulocytosis, cyclical neutropenia and anaemia. These conditions affect the capacity of the oral mucosa to heal and resist infection. Ulcers are most probably precipitated by trauma and therefore occur more commonly on non-keratinized mucosal surfaces. Ulcerative stomatitis can also occur in uraemia, in heavy metal poisoning especially with gold, in uncontrolled diabetes and as a complication following the use of cytotoxic drugs such as aminopterin and methotrexate. In these cases the ulcers are probably the result of cytopenia rather than an idiosyncrasy to the drug.

The treatment of such ulceration should be directed mainly at the elimination of the aetiological factor. However, palliative treatment by the application of a surface covering with Orabase and the administration of lozenges containing a surface anaesthetic for the control of pain may be helpful.

9. Oral Manifestations of Sexually Transmitted Disease

D. A. McGowan, D. Stenhouse and C. E. Renson

Oral manifestations of sexually transmitted disease must be constantly borne in mind, not least because of the risk of spread of infection by this route to the examining clinician. The lesions will go unrecognized unless the suspicion of sexually transmitted disease prompts an examination of the mouth as well as more obvious sites and unless this possible explanation for oral symptoms is remembered. The use of rubber finger stalls or gloves in examination of all patients with oral ulceration is a sensible precaution.

Syphilis

Syphilis at all its stages can exhibit dental or oral mucosal abnormalities. Congenital syphilis can cause disruption of morphogenesis of the teeth which develop in the first year of life. Most obviously affected, therefore, are the upper central incisors, 'Hutchinson's incisors' (Figure 9.1,a and b). The incisal edge notching is less prominent in the second example but the barrel-shaped crowns are well marked in both. The molar crowns may also be affected, the so-called 'Moon's molars', or more descriptively termed 'mulberry molars'. These changes may be evident as part of Hutchinson's Triad which also includes interstitial keratitis and deafness. Other characteristics of congenital syphilis such as saddle nose deformity, frontal bossing and rhagades are shown in Figure 9.2 and the use of an old black and white illustration indicates the rarity of the condition in recent times. Modern obstetric practice of routine screening of antenatal patients must take the credit for the virtual elimination of this stigmatic appearance.

Primary Syphilis

Acquired syphilis may cause oral lesions at all three stages of the disease. The chancre of primary syphilis can occur in or around the oral cavity, most commonly on the tongue or lips. As elsewhere the chancre presents as a raised nodular lesion 2 to 3 cm in diameter with an ulcerated or crusted centre (Figure 9.3), and there may be associated

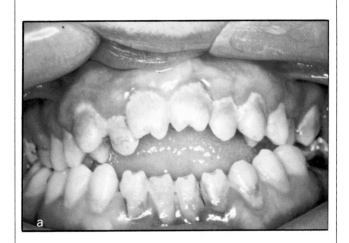
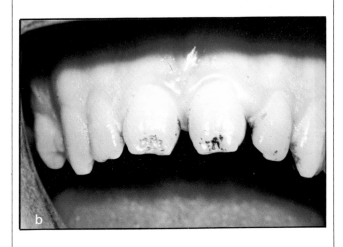

Figure 9.1. *(a) and (b) Congenital syphilis: Hutchinson's incisors. The incisal edge notching is less prominent in (b) but the barrel-shaped crowns are well marked in both examples.*

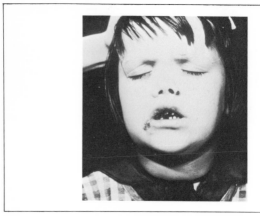

Figure 9.2. *Congenital syphilis: rhagades are infected, painful fissures at the angles of the mouth. This figure also illustrates the saddle nose deformity and frontal bossing.*

Figure 9.3. *(a) and (b) Syphilis: a primary chancre appears three to four weeks after infection. The site may be the lips (as in these two examples) or the tip of the tongue.*

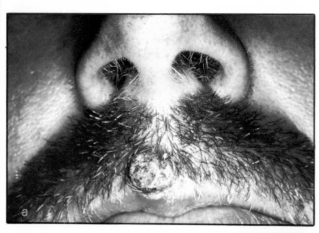

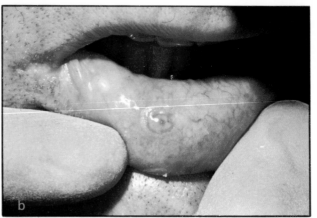

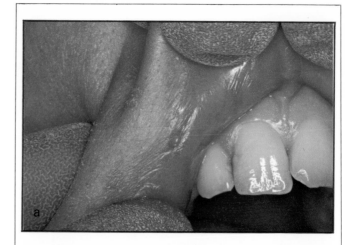

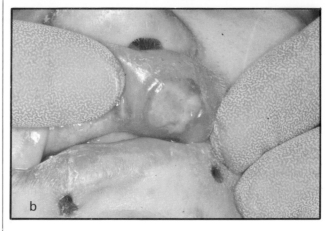

Figure 9.4. *(a) Syphilis: secondary syphilitic lesions of the lip. The lesion in (b) takes the form of the 'mucous patch'.*

painless rubbery enlargement of the regional lymph nodes. The primary lesions are highly infective and spirochaetes can be isolated from their surface.

Secondary Syphilis

Secondary syphilis may cause oral ulceration. The ulcers may closely simulate recurrent aphthous ulcers, or the ulceration caused by Behcet's syndrome, erythema multiforme or herpes simplex (Chapter 8). Figure 9.4 shows secondary syphilitic ulcers of the lip. In Figure 9.4a, the apparent innocence of the small lesion is illustrated and the danger to the unwary clinician is stressed. A more characteristic mucous patch and neighbouring skin lesions can be seen in Figure 9.4b. The appearance of a split papule is shown in Figure 9.5 and is regarded as characteristic of the secondary lesion. Another syphilitic ulcer of the tongue is seen in Figure 9.6 which could not be

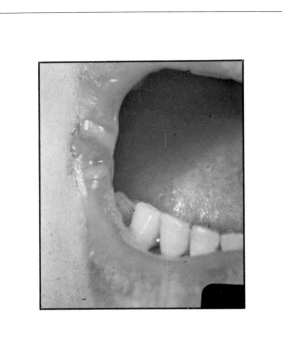

Figure 9.5. *Syphilis: the split papule appearance at the angle of the mouth sometimes occurs in secondary syphilis.*

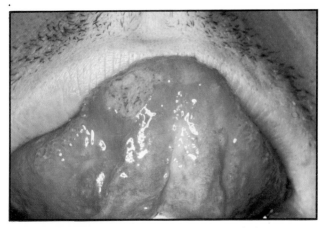

Figure 9.6. *Syphilis: a syphilitic ulcer of the tongue which resembles a simple traumatic ulcer or a recurrent aphthous ulcer.*

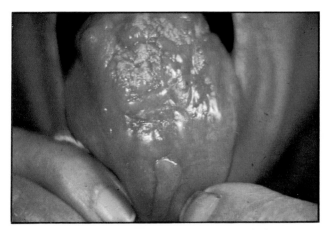

Figure 9.7. *Tertiary syphilis: a gumma of the tongue. Note the rounded outline with soft punched-out edges.*

distinguished from a simple traumatic ulcer or a recurrent aphthous ulcer without further investigation. Generally the mucous patch is shallow, well demarcated by an erythematous border and has a pale grey sloughing centre. These lesions are also rich in spirochaetes and must be handled with caution. Although oral manifestations are rare without skin involvement, the latter may not be readily apparent on the visible skin surfaces of an outpatient.

Tertiary Syphilis

Thanks to the use of modern antibiotics in earlier stages tertiary syphilis is now extremely uncommon. A gumma may arise in the mouth as in any other part of the body. It is essentially a granulomatous proliferation which will destroy tissue locally. Figure 9.7 shows a gumma of the tongue while Figure 9.8 vividly illustrates the destructive properties of a gumma which has produced perforation of the hard palate. Another manifestation of tertiary syphilis is a gross leukoplakia which affects the dorsum of the tongue (Figure 9.9). This is a well recognized premalignant lesion, and any ulceration or other change in character is an indication for immediate biopsy to exclude squamous cell carcinoma.

Figure 9.8. *Tertiary syphilis: a gumma of the palate. Necrosis has caused a perforation of the bone and a typical round punched-out hole.*

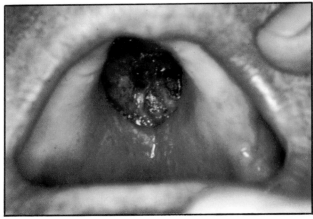

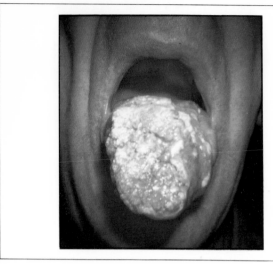

Figure 9.9. *Tertiary syphilis: gross leukoplakia affecting the dorsum of the tongue.*

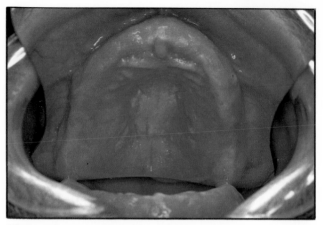

Figure 9.11. *Reiter's disease: an irregular erythema confined to the alveolar ridge.*

Figure 9.12. *Reiter's disease: confluent patches of acutely erythematous mucosa in the lining of the cheek.*

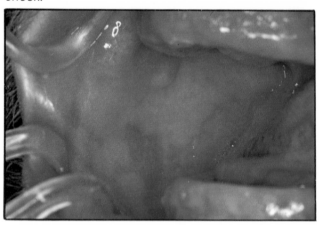

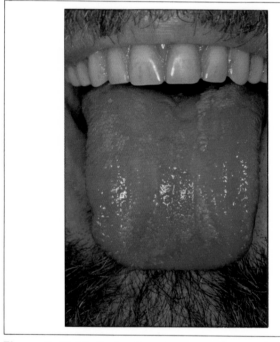

Figure 9.10. *Reiter's disease: note the erythema along the lateral margins of the tongue.*

taken from the same patient. Figure 9.10 shows the appearance of the tongue with a central area of normal or atrophic papillae merging with areas of erythema particularly along the lateral margins. Figure 9.11 shows the edentulous palate with an irregular erythema confined to the alveolar ridge. The appearance of the cheek in Figure 9.12 is similar to that of the palate and tongue with confluent patches of acutely erythematous mucosa standing out in sharp contrast to the normal pink mucous membrane of this area.

Reiter's Disease

Reiter's disease consists of acute urethritis, arthritis, and conjunctivitis with variable skin or oral involvement. It predominantly affects young males and is generally held to be sexually transmitted. Figures 9.10, 9.11 and 9.12 are

Herpetic Ulceration

Oral herpetic ulceration may also arise as a sexually transmitted disease though this is a rare association. An example is illustrated in Figure 9.13 (a and b).

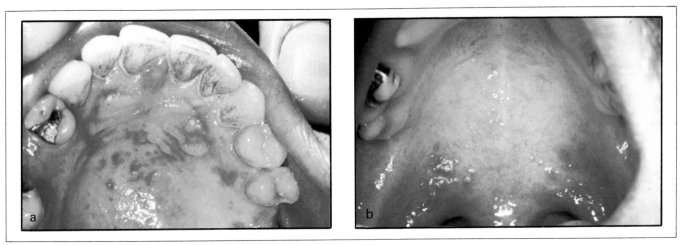

Figure 9.13. *(a) and (b) Oral herpetic ulceration may also arise as a sexually transmitted lesion.*

10. The Salivary Glands

G. R. Seward

Complaints related to the salivary glands tend to fall into the following groups: an acute swelling, a recurrent swelling, a persistent swelling, a dry mouth or excessive salivation.

Acute Swelling

Mumps

Mumps is the most common cause of acute swelling of the salivary glands. Most general practitioners will have handled patients affected during the regular epidemics of this disease. It is worth remembering, however, that the disease is very variable. Some patients may be very ill and suffer from meningoencephalitis, pancreatitis or orchitis. Indeed, one or the other of these manifestations may overshadow the salivary gland enlargement making for diagnostic difficulties. At the other extreme the patient may feel quite well, but will have an enlargement of one or more salivary glands; sometimes only the submandibular glands (Figure 10.1) or even just the cervical lymph nodes. Other viruses, such as Adenovirus and Coxsackie A, may also be a cause of acute parotitis. Where there is doubt about the diagnosis and where accuracy is important the determination of S and V antibody titres in the patient's serum on two occasions, two to three weeks apart, will confirm or refute the diagnosis.

Acute Suppurative Parotitis

Acute suppurative parotitis now occurs more often as a sequel to chronic duct obstruction than as a postoperative complication in the debilitated patient. Such attacks must be distinguished from acute submasseteric abscess and acute infections of the pre-auricular or upper deep cervical lymph nodes. In acute parotitis, if the masseters are palpated while the jaws are clenched and released, the muscle may be distinguished anterior to the swelling. With an acute submasseteric abscess the swelling is anterior to the parotid. The absence of a purulent discharge at the papilla

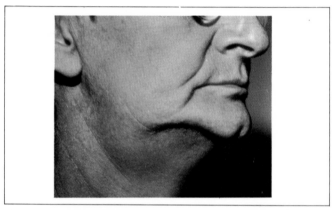

Figure 10.1. *A patient with enlargement of one submandibular salivary gland. The gland had been swollen for 14 days but the patient had not felt unwell in any other way. Serological tests confirmed the diagnosis of mumps and several contacts developed the disease.*

when the gland is gently massaged helps to distinguish acute lymph node infections from parotitis.

Prompt antibiotic treatment makes the need for surgical drainage of a parotid abscess a comparatively rare occurrence these days. Such cases should be investigated further after the acute infection has subsided to try to establish the underlying reason for the attack.

Recurrent Enlargement

Broadly speaking recurrent enlargement may amount to recurrent swelling at mealtimes, which is caused by duct obstruction, and recurrent episodes of swelling lasting several days and which are caused by recurrent subacute infections occurring as a result of chronic retention of secretions.

Calculi

The most frequent cause of recurrent enlargement at mealtimes is a calculus. While submandibular calculi are by far the most common (Figure 10.2), parotid calculi are found more frequently than is generally believed (Figure 10.3). The reason is that there are difficulties associated with displaying small parotid calculi by plain radiography. Many are only picked up by sialography and, even then, some special skill and experience of this technique may be necessary if calculi are not to be missed. Diagnosis is important in these cases as parotid calculi are more amenable to treatment than most causes of parotid disease. When calculi are identified a careful, systematic approach to their removal should be made, based on a proper regard for the anatomy of the part.

Sublingual and minor salivary gland calculi have been recognized with increasing frequency in recent years, and can be the underlying cause of swelling of the respective glands.

Strictures

Strictures of the ducts of the major glands are another cause of mealtime swelling. They may result from ulceration around a calculus, or traumatic damage to the duct. Bilateral parotid duct strictures which occur opposite the anterior or posterior border of the mandible may be autoimmune in origin, but do not seem to be related to Sjögren's disease. The glandular swelling resulting from posterior strictures produces limitation of jaw opening and pain on mastication, and so mimics temporomandibular joint disease. As the deep part of the gland is involved there is no visible swelling. Duct implantation, grafting and bouginage can be used to treat strictures.

Trauma

Acute trauma to a duct papilla will result in an ulcer around the duct orifice (Figure 10.4) and mealtime swelling of the gland until the ulcer heals and the oedema subsides. Chronic trauma from a sharp tooth or a denture will result in chronic papillary stenosis which can be cured only by a papillotomy with careful suture of the duct lining to the oral mucosa.

Neoplasms and Cysts

Benign neoplasms and cysts which press on the ducts, or malignant neoplasms which come to invade the ducts are occasional causes of duct obstruction.

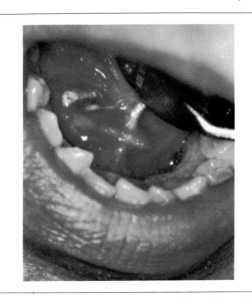

Figure 10.2. *A submandibular calculus ulcerating through into the mouth. These calculi are spontaneously discharged in this way. The duct opening is too small to let them pass.*

Figure 10.3. *The parotid duct opening is larger than the submandibular and small calculi may protrude from it.*

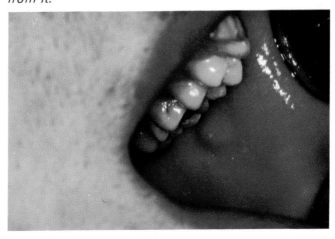

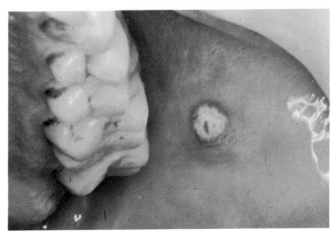

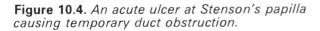

Figure 10.4. *An acute ulcer at Stenson's papilla causing temporary duct obstruction.*

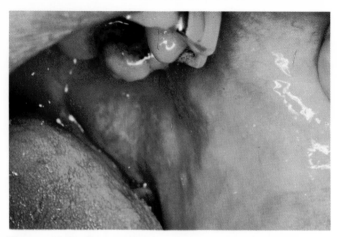

Figure 10.5. *Generalized salivary gland enlargement caused by antithyroid agent. The patient had difficulty in closing his mouth because of enlargement of buccal and retromolar glands.*

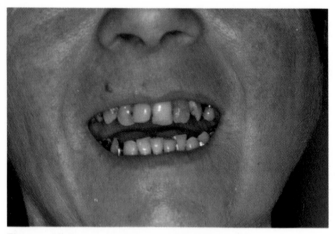

Figure 10.6. *Limitation of opening of the mouth and enlargement of the parotid gland caused by squamous cell carcinoma of the deep part of the parotid which was invading the mandible. There is as yet no facial paralysis.*

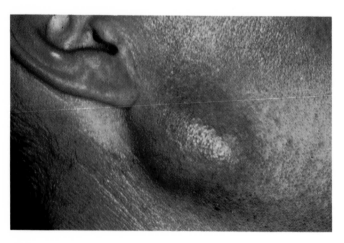

Sialoadenitis and Sialectasis

Most of these aetiological factors may be the underlying cause of an acute suppurative sialoadenitis, or recurrent attacks of subacute infection. In these cases there is chronic incomplete obstruction with duct dilatation, but the obstruction may not be severe enough to cause regular mealtime swelling.

The sialographic appearance of punctate sialectasis, that is, numerous small globular cavities filled with the contrast medium occurring at the periphery of the gland, is probably in the adult a non-specific finding. It can be found in some cases of Sjögren's syndrome, following therapeutic irradiation of a gland, or even following chronic obstruction with ascending infection. However, the appearance is also characteristic of a condition which mostly causes symptoms in childhood. Almost all young children who have recurrent subacute infections of the parotid glands have this sialographic appearance. A few will be found to have a calculus, for calculi in children are more common than is generally recognized.

Treatment

The attacks should be treated with penicillin orally to limit damage to the gland, but the final outcome is favourable. Katzen (1969) has shown in a linear study that spontaneous remission by 15 years of age is the usual course. A sialogram frequently induces a remission and can be considered a diagnostic and a therapeutic manoeuvre. A few patients produce multiple small calculi in these cavities which may come down the ducts and cause obstruction. The disease does not seem to progress to Sjögren's syndrome in the adult.

Other Causes of Recurrent Swelling

Uncommon causes of recurrent swelling are allergic parotitis and the effects of certain drugs. In both cases there is no suggestion of ascending infection. Clinical evidence in favour of an allergic parotitis is a past history of other allergic reactions such as urticarial rashes or hay fever. In some cases a cause—effect relationship to contact with an allergen may be established.

A number of drugs produce enlargement of the salivary glands. For example, phenylbutazone, isoprenaline and phenothiazine derivatives, iodine and most of the drugs used to treat thyrotoxicosis, such as thiouracil (Figure 10.5). Drugs which reduce salivary secretion and steroids

Figure 10.7. *(Left) A parotid pleomorphic adenoma producing the characteristic lobulated firm swelling at the lower pole.*

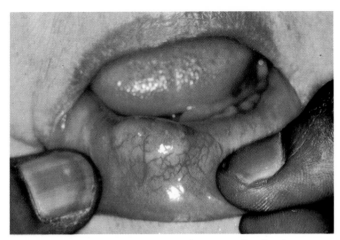

Figure 10.8. *A pleomorphic adenoma in the lower lip. Notice the enlarged vessels over the surface. Pleomorphic adenomas of the minor salivary glands are often misdiagnosed. In particular, palatal ones are mistaken for abscesses and incised.*

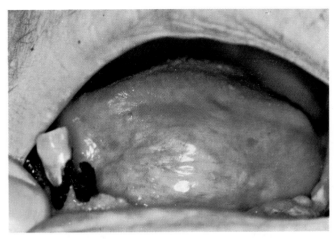

Figure 10.9. *An adenocystic carcinoma of the left submandibular salivary gland invading the sublingual tissues and tongue. The slowly enlarging neoplasm was tolerated by the patient until it was inoperable.*

may also predispose patients to attacks of ascending infection.

Diabetics and patients addicted to unusual diets, especially protein deficient diets, may suffer from a more sustained enlargement of the salivary glands.

Persistent Swellings

Persistent enlargement, particularly persistent localized enlargement is suggestive of a neoplasm. However, other causes may be encountered. Sarcoid, Hodgkin's disease, tuberculosis and chronic infection of lymph nodes within the gland, for instance, because of frequent sore throats, are infrequent causes, some of which may be identified only after a biopsy. A careful history and physical examination may differentiate neoplasms and hamartomas of associated tissues, such as neurofibromas, haemangiomas and lipomas, provided the possibility is considered. Neurofibromas elsewhere, signs of increased vascularity of the part and deposits of fat in the neck may be suggestive signs in such cases.

Neoplasms

True salivary gland neoplasms can present considerable problems. Where there are obvious signs of malignancy such as fixation, invasion of the mandible, or loss of function of adjacent nerves decisions on management are not too difficult (Figure 10.6). Where the patient has had a nodular, firm mass for a number of years without signs or symptoms suggestive of invasion a pleomorphic adenoma is the likely diagnosis (Figures 10.7 and 10.8). One, or possibly more, rounded, smooth, soft or fluctuant

swellings in the middle-aged or elderly man are likely to be papillary-cystadenoma lymphomatosum.

Management

Difficulty in management stems mainly from the existence of certain slowly growing yet invasive neoplasms. The mucoepidermoid carcinoma and the adenocystic carcinoma can present this problem (Figure 10.9). They may present clinically as a modest swelling which has been present for several years and may closely resemble the pleomorphic adenoma. However, a technique of excision which is adequate to ensure removal of the latter is quite likely to leave residual tumour in the case of a mucoepidermoid carcinoma and would be quite inadequate for an adenocystic carcinoma. The latter is particularly sinister in the way in which it penetrates for long distances along the perineural lymphatics, and in its ability to penetrate bone without inducing radiographically detectable bone resorption.

Mikulicz's Disease

Bilateral enlargement of the glands is seen in Mikulicz's disease (Figure 10.10) which is now viewed as a variant of Sjögren's syndrome and is autoimmune in aetiology. Some cases, however, exhibit a nodular enlargement which may resemble either a neoplasm or sarcoid on clinical examination.

Dry Mouth

Sjögren's syndrome is probably the most common cause of a truly dry mouth. Clinically, cases have a dry mouth,

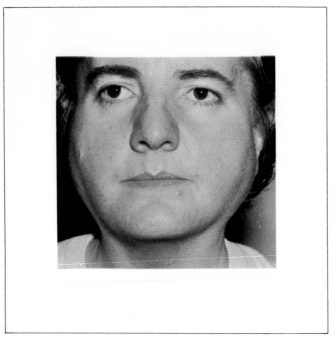

Figure 10.10. *Mikulicz's disease. Chronic enlargement of both parotid glands in a patient with dry mouth and eyes. Tests were positive for rheumatoid factor, antinuclear factor and salivary duct antibodies. Histological confirmation of Sjögren's disease was obtained from a labial gland biopsy.*

dry eyes and rheumatoid arthritis in varying combination but many other disturbances are now recognized as part of the syndrome. Obstructive symptoms caused by strictures or calculi and attacks of ascending infection as a result of reduced salivary flow, may add to the patient's salivary troubles. Nothing will increase the patient's salivary flow. However, frequent sips of water at mealtimes and a lubricant for lips and cheeks between meals may help to reduce the patient's discomfort.

Excessive Salivation

The usual cause is a failure of the patient to deal adequately with a normal salivary flow. Difficulty in swallowing, oral ulcers, or abnormalities of the tongue or lips may result in this complaint. The presence of new dentures in the mouth is frequently associated with difficulty in managing the saliva. Some newly edentulous patients become aware of their parotid secretions for the first time, note its taste and complain of a discharge from the cheeks.

Too much or too little saliva may be a complaint of the mentally disturbed. Here inspection of the oral cavity will reveal no abnormal findings.

Reference
Katzen, M., *S. Afr. Med. J.,* 1969, **7**, 37.

11. Diseases of the Jaws

D. A. McGowan

Two special features complicate the diagnosis of disease in the maxillo-facial region. The first is the existence of a range of pathological conditions arising directly from the teeth and the dental formative tissues. The second is the unique anatomical structure composed of bone covered largely by a relatively thin layer of mucoperiosteum pierced by calcified structures.

The field is too wide to allow systematic treatment in this chapter so only a few conditions will be described to draw attention to some areas of diagnostic confusion.

The presence in the jaws of unerupted teeth or retained dental fragments is a relatively frequent cause of symptoms in patients who are apparently edentulous. Such patients tend to shed their connection with the dental profession with their teeth, and are more likely to seek help from their medical practitioner even for purely oral symptoms.

Symptoms

Pain, bad taste or more bizarre complaints such as dentures 'wearing through to the bone' can arise from the presence of such teeth. When chronic inflammation is marked, the appearance may closely resemble a neoplastic ulcer, but dental radiographic examination will readily identify the underlying cause.

The patient in Figure 11.1 has a retained malpositioned upper right canine tooth, the blackened carious surface of which can be easily seen. A smaller retained root fragment is also visible in the left premolar area. Such fragments have a characteristic flinty-hard feel on probing which helps to distinguish them from exposed bone. Retained teeth become exposed in the course of time as resorption of the alveolar ridges progresses. Removal of these teeth produces complete relief of the symptoms.

Dental abscesses usually produce swelling and discharge within the mouth, but occasionally the infection may track externally and produce a sinus in the overlying skin. Figure 11.2a shows such a lesion. This site is characteristic of a sinus arising from a lower molar and Figure 11.2b shows the cause—a grossly decayed lower first molar.

External sinuses such as these have been mistaken for basal cell carcinoma, and even treated as such. Removal of this young man's tooth allowed the lesion to heal in a few months (Figure 11.2c).

Chronic Diseases

Localized Symptoms of Systemic Disease

Chronic infectious diseases such as tuberculosis or actinomycosis may present in the cervico-mandibular region. These can be confused with abscesses of dental origin, but the absence of an obvious cause in the mouth or persistence of swelling after tooth extraction should arouse suspicion. The patient in Figure 11.3 has a tuberculous lymph node infection. Actinomycosis can present a very similar appearance and a raised, discrete, purplish, nodular swelling surrounded by normal looking skin is particularly characteristic. The classical description of multiple sinuses discharging sulphur granules is less com-

Figure 11.1. *Edentulous upper jaw showing buried tooth on right and retained root on left.*

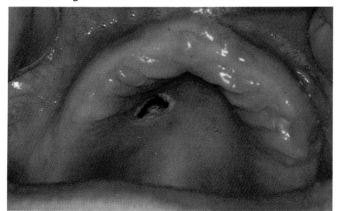

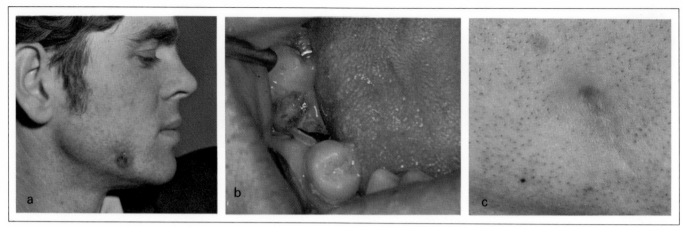

Figure 11.2. *(a) External sinus caused by dental abscess of lower molar. (b) Grossly decayed lower molar which caused sinus shown in (a). (c) Healing area of skin six months after extraction of lower molar shown in (b).*

Figure 11.3. *Tuberculous abscess.*

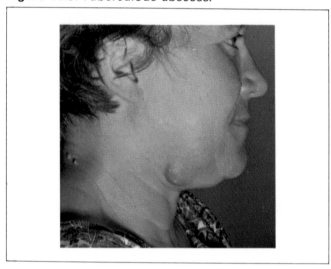

Figure 11.4. *Exfoliating molar tooth caused by destruction of supporting bone associated with histiocytosis-X.*

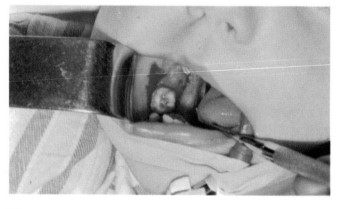

monly fulfilled nowadays.

In the same way, osteomyelitis of the mandible is usually found in a much less dramatic form than in the pre-antibiotic era. A chronic severe dull ache associated with numbness of the lip on the affected side is the most likely presenting symptom.

Apparently trivial localized symptoms in the mouth may be the first recognizable effect of serious systemic disease. The child in Figure 11.4 was brought to the dentist because his mother noticed increasing looseness of his right lower first permanent molar. Radiographic examination showed complete destruction of the supporting bone and biopsy established a diagnosis of histiocytosis-X.

Figure 11.5 shows a secondary deposit in the anterior mandibular region from an adrenal medullary neuroblastoma. The complaint was of swelling and mobility and displacement of the teeth.

The expansion of buccal and lingual sides of the jaw should be particularly noted, as this is a feature more frequently associated with tumours in the jaws than with cysts which are much more common lesions.

A typical dental cyst is shown in Figure 11.6. There are many different types of cysts of the jaws, but those arising as a long-term sequel of dental infection are the most common. These have an excellent prognosis and surgical enucleation (Figures 11.7 and 11.8) is almost always curative. Some of the other types, however, are more difficult to eliminate and more radical surgery may be necessary.

These lesions produce few symptoms until they become large and produce noticeable expansion of the bone—usually on the buccal side. They are only painful if infection or pathological fracture ensues.

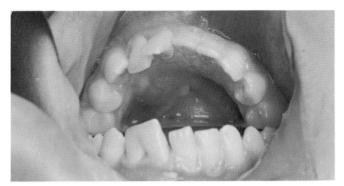

Figure 11.5. *Swelling of the lower anterior region (seen in a mirror) which proved to be a secondary from an adrenal medullary neuroblastoma.*

Figure 11.6. *Buccal swelling caused by a dental cyst.*

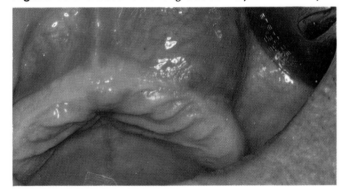

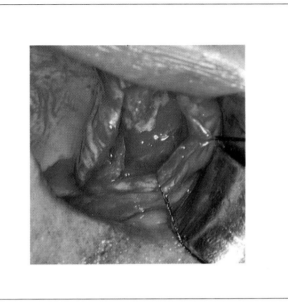

Figure 11.7. *Dental cyst — cavity left after enucleation.*

Bone Diseases

Systemic bone diseases affecting the jaws may produce special problems especially when tooth extraction is necessary. Even trivial breaches in the overlying mucosa, perhaps associated with denture trauma, may initiate chronic infection in the abnormal bone leading to localized sequestration or chronic discharge.

Paget's Disease

Paget's disease may affect either mandible or maxilla alone or as a part of a general skeletal involvement. The characteristic enlargement is shown in Figures 11.9 and 11.10 and the rich vascular supply to the bone is evident in Figure 11.9. This creates problems with bleeding after tooth extraction. In addition, the teeth are affected in that excessive cementum is laid down on the root surface. The classical increase in cranial diameter is mirrored in the mouth by enlargement of the alveolar ridges—leading to a need for increasingly large dentures as well as hats!

Similar problems arise in osteopetrosis when a particularly recalcitrant form of bone infection may occur.

Figure 11.8. *Dental cyst — flap sutured.*

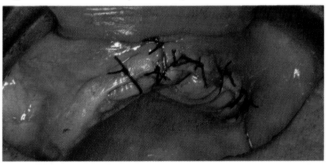

Figure 11.9. *Paget's disease of the maxilla.*

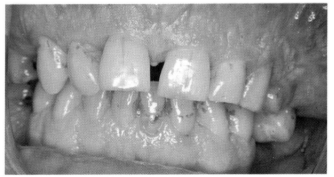

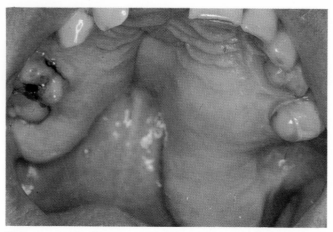

Figure 11.10. *Paget's disease of the maxilla showing gross enlargement of the left maxillary tuberosity.*

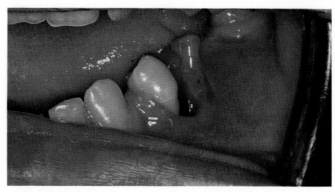

Figure 11.12. *Fracture of the mandible. Note the occlusion of the posterior teeth but separation of the anterior teeth.*

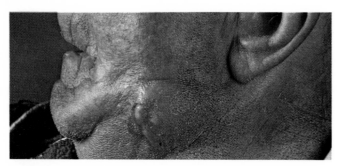

Figure 11.11. *Radionecrosis of the mandible with pathological fracture and external discharge.*

Figure 11.13. *Tetanus — 'risus sardonicus'.*

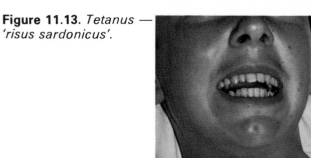

Radionecrosis

Therapeutic radiation to the jaws with consequent reduction in salivary secretion can cause rampant dental caries, though this is commonly prevented by extraction of teeth before treatment. Radionecrosis of the jaws, though less common now because of more sophisticated radiotherapeutic techniques, presents a major problem in some patients following treatment for malignant disease in the mouth.

Tissue breakdown may lead to a salivary fistula and the area usually affected is shown in Figure 11.11. This patient had also sustained a pathological fracture of the mandible. Successful treatment of such cases may require extensive grafting procedures to provide coverage with better vascularized tissue.

Early treatment of caries in retained teeth and scrupulous maintenance or withdrawal of dentures may help to prevent the establishment of radionecrosis.

Restriction of Mandibular Movement

Figure 11.12 shows a fracture of the mandible in the left premolar area of a young girl, who had injured herself in a fall, during an epileptic fit. Though such an obvious breach in continuity is not always apparent, careful clinical examination will reveal evidence of most jaw fractures. Pain may not be a prominent feature, except on movement, but derangement of the occlusion of the teeth is easily seen when the tooth bearing areas are involved and the patient is usually conscious of the fact that he cannot bite normally. If the normal range of mandibular movements can be performed without pain or restriction, and if no pain is produced on bilateral finger pressure over the angles, then the presence of a mandibular fracture is unlikely. Radiographic examination is essential for definitive diagnosis in such injuries, but clinical examination alone may allow early diagnosis and prompt referral for treatment.

There are many possible causes of limitation of mandibular movement. One of the commonest, apart from trauma, is the restriction of opening which occurs as a consequence of infection around the lower wisdom teeth in a young adult. Though antibiotics are of great assistance in the treatment of such infections, local dental measures are of at least equal importance. Other rare causes, such as tetanus (Figure 11.13), must not be forgotten.

Conclusion

Though dental surgeons are specially trained to recognize and treat diseases of the jaws as well as those of the teeth, most patients with such problems will consult first with their doctor—the person to whom they turn automatically when they feel ill. Close cooperation between the professions is vital to the provision of a proper service.

Section 4
Neoplasms in the Mouth

12. Tumours and Tumour-like Lesions

C. C. Rachanis

The spectrum of tissues to be found in different parts of the mouth includes keratinizing and non-keratinizing epithelium, a variety of mesodermal components ranging from bone to lymphoid tissue, and a rich salivary tissue component. Therefore, the majority of the neoplasms arising from the oral tissues have exact counterparts in other regions of the body, and when they occur in the mouth they are no different in essentials to equivalent lesions elsewhere. However, the mouth does give rise to one group of tumours, peculiar to the jaws, which arise from the tooth-forming apparatus; these latter will be dealt with in the next chapter.

Tumour-like Masses

Proliferative lesions occurring in the mouth may be true neoplasms, although a number of different lesions arising from the oral tissues are tumour-like inflammatory masses which, clinically, may resemble neoplasms rather closely. Among these are the pyogenic granuloma, the fibro-epithelial polyp, the fibrous epulis, irritative hyperplasia ('denture' granuloma), and the so-called 'peripheral giant cell granuloma'. Fortunately, true neoplasms of the mouth are relatively uncommon. Many of the lesions to be discussed under the heading of benign tumours are now considered to be developmental malformations rather than true neoplasms. With a few exceptions they are totally innocent, without malignant potential and without therapeutic problems. Clinically, they may be confused with malignant neoplasms, especially if traumatized and secondarily infected.

Pyogenic Granuloma

This lesion of the oral mucosa appears clinically as an elevated, pedunculated or sessile swelling bright red in colour and varying in diameter from several millimetres to a centimetre or more. Sites of occurrence are the lips, tongue, buccal mucosa and gingiva (Figure 12.1).

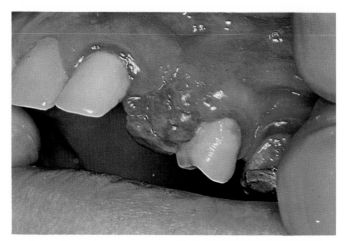

Figure 12.1. *Pyogenic granuloma situated in upper left canine region but associated with the first premolar tooth.*

The surface may be covered by a white or yellow slough depending upon the degree of superimposed purulent inflammation. The lesion represents a reaction to localized irritation which is characterized by extensive proliferation of granulation tissue. This tissue is easily traumatized, its surface ulcerated and secondarily infected with oral pyogenic bacteria.

Treatment consists of surgical excision and the removal of all sources of trauma in the area, e.g. sharp or rough edges on teeth and/or restorations. Incomplete excision may result in recurrence of the lesion.

Fibroepithelial Polyp

This very common benign lesion of the oral mucosa is often incorrectly referred to as a 'papilloma'. Whereas the intra-oral papilloma appears to be a benign neoplasm of epithelial tissue, the fibroepithelial polyp is composed of reparative fibrous tissue, covered by a thin layer of

62

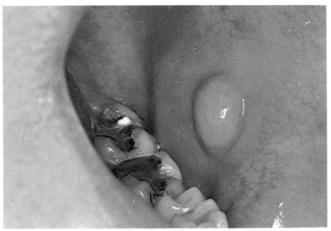

Figure 12.2. *Fibroepithelial polyp presenting as a smooth, soft, sessile, pink swelling on buccal mucosa, level with the occlusal surfaces of the teeth on closure.*

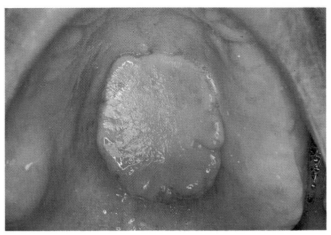

Figure 12.3. *Fibroepithelial polyp of hard palate assuming flattened leaf-like shape under a denture.*

Figure 12.4. *Localized hyperplasia of gingival tissue associated with chronic periodontal disease.*

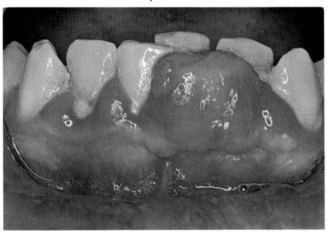

stratified squamous epithelium. It may be the result of irritation or trauma and may appear anywhere in the mouth (Figure 12.2). It usually has a smooth surface but occasionally it may be slightly papillary in form. Its shape and size vary considerably. It may be pedunculated or broad-based and sometimes a leaf-like lesion may be found on the denture-bearing area of the mucosa (Figure 12.3). It is treated by simple excision.

Fibrous Epulis

This is a lesion occurring on the gingiva (Figure 12.4), and is probably a localized hyperplasia of the connective tissue following trauma and/or inflammation in the area. Tissue alterations comprising the reparative stages of the inflammatory reaction probably continue, with the formation of an excessive amount of connective tissue. It is often incorrectly referred to as a 'fibroma'. This lesion is not well differentiated from the previously described fibroepithelial polyp.

Treatment is by conservative excision with special attention being paid to the restoration of a healthy gingival contour.

Irritative Hyperplasia ('Denture' Hyperplasia or Granuloma)

Irritative hyperplasia occurs in edentulous or partly edentulous mouths, arising from the mucosal tissue of the edentulous ridge, adjacent buccal mucosa (Figure 12.5) or lingual sulcus. The lesion is an inflammatory hyperplasia in response to a local irritation, invariably the over-extended flange of a denture. Clinically, it is frequently

Figure 12.5. *Hyperplasia of buccal mucosa caused by chronic irritation from flange of ill-fitting lower denture.*

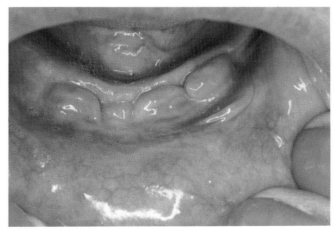

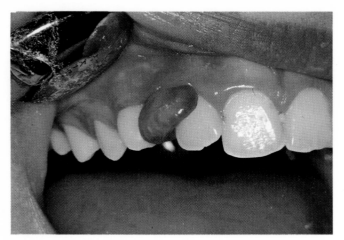

Figure 12.6. *Peripheral reparative giant cell granuloma presenting on labial maxillary gingiva, from interdental papilla, extending almost to occlusal surfaces of teeth.*

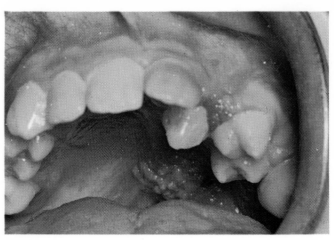

Figure 12.7. *Cauliflower-like surface of sessile papilloma of the palate.*

seen as an elongated raised mass of firm, pink or red tissue, which may show a cleft caused by the denture flange. This may become ulcerated and painful because of persistent irritation. Although the clinical appearance and relationship of the denture may suggest the diagnosis, it is most important to remember that squamous cell carcinoma may arise in close contact with a denture. Therefore, it is imperative that malignant neoplasia be considered and ruled out, if necessary, by biopsy.

Treatment will usually include removal of the excessive fibrotic tissue and remodelling of the denture, or the construction of new well-fitting dentures.

Peripheral Reparative Giant Cell Granuloma

This is a benign tumour-like lesion of the gingiva within which multinucleated giant cells are prominent. It occurs with equal frequency in the maxillary and mandibular gingiva, usually in the region of the interdental papilla (Figure 12.6); occasionally it may arise in an edentulous area. It is relatively rare. The lesion is considered to be an unusually proliferative response of the tissue to some form of local irritation or trauma.

Clinically, the peripheral reparative giant cell granuloma presents as a slowly growing, sessile or pedunculated firm mass with a smooth shiny surface, varying in colour from pink to purple-red. If traumatized it bleeds easily. As the lesion increases in size it may exert pressure on the adjacent teeth with displacement and resultant malocclusion, or it may grow sufficiently to interfere with mastication. Unless traumatized surface ulceration is minimal and pain is not usually a feature. Being a soft tissue lesion the underlying alveolar bone is rarely

involved, although radiographs, especially of the more rapidly growing lesions, may show slight bone resorption.

Treatment consists of surgical excision, without sacrifice of the adjacent teeth, but many recommend curettage of the surface of the underlying bone. With incomplete removal the lesion may recur.

Papilloma

Several tumours and tumour-like lesions appear clinically as 'papillomatous lesions', but the term papilloma should be used specifically for a benign lesion of the epithelium with a branching filiform structure and a fine connective tissue core. Papilloma describes the macroscopic appearance, i.e. papillary or cauliflower-like. Structurally the papilloma resembles the viral wart of the skin, but viral inclusions are rarely, if ever, demonstrated.

Clinically, the papilloma appears as a fine, white, exophytic lesion arising from the oral mucosa. On rare occasions it may grow inwards when it has the appearance of a slightly raised nodular pink mass. The degree of keratinization of the papilloma probably influences the colour. It usually has a narrow pedicle but may have a broad base. The size varies from several millimetres to several centimetres in diameter, but the majority are usually less than one centimetre. Although it may arise from any part of the oral mucosa the usual sites are the dorsum of the tongue, the buccal and labial mucosa, and the palate (Figure 12.7). The papilloma is usually single but multiple papillomata may be seen.

Simple excision is sufficient treatment. In contrast to papillomata of the respiratory tract and bladder there is little tendency to recurrence. The large papillomata may

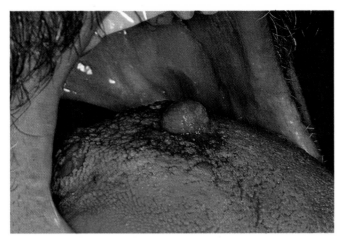

Figure 12.8. *Pedunculated fibroma on dorsum of posterior third of tongue.*

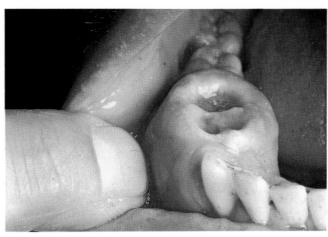

Figure 12.9. *Large fibroma of gingiva occupying premolar region and showing impression of occlusal surfaces.*

be difficult to distinguish clinically from the papillary variety of well differentiated squamous cell carcinoma, early verrucous carcinoma or the papillary form of leukoplakia. Because of these doubts all papillary lesions, no matter how small, should be examined histologically.

Pleomorphic Adenoma

A pleomorphic adenoma (so-called 'mixed' salivary tumour), of salivary gland tissue is a common neoplasm of the parotid gland and occasionally it may be found arising from mucous glands (minor salivary glands) of the oral mucosa. Clinically, it appears as a small, spherical, freely movable mass beneath the surface of the mucosa. An adenoma increases slowly in size and if not removed may develop into a mass of up to about 2 cm in diameter. It may occur in the palate, tongue, lips and cheek. A pleomorphic adenoma is a well-circumscribed spongy mass expanding outwards from the mucosal corium; or it may present as a smooth firm nodule beneath the mucosa. When large the tumour projects above the mucosal surface.

Treatment consists of surgical excision including a narrow margin of uninvolved tissue to avoid the possibility of recurrence. In spite of this, there may be recurrences because of the often multifocal origin of this tumour.

Fibroma

The true fibroma is a relatively uncommon benign tumour of fibrous connective tissue. Clinically, the fibroma is usually a small, discrete spherical to ovoid nodule of firm consistency varying from a soft, rubbery pliable mass to an extremely hard, unyielding nodule. It is usually covered with mucosa presenting a shiny surface. The size varies from a pea to the size of a golf ball in rare instances, and it may be pedunculated and easily movable or broad-based and relatively immovable. Its colour varies from a light pink to a deep pink red. The fibroma may occur anywhere in the mouth and is painless (Figures 12.8 and 12.9). It is resistant to mechanical irritation and usually does not become ulcerated or infected, but in the very large tumours secondary inflammatory alterations may be a feature.

In a few instances the oral fibroma appears to be developmental in origin; tending to occur bilaterally and being most commonly observed on the maxillary tuberosities attached to the gingiva ('symmetrical fibroma'). Extensive gingival fibromatosis or 'elephantiasis gingivae' develops as the deciduous teeth erupt and may be sufficiently extensive to cover the crowns of the teeth. This condition must be distinguished from other forms of gingival enlargement or hyperplasia, e.g. phenytoin gingival hyperplasia. Gingival inflammation tends to be minimal in gingival fibromatosis. Treatment is by radical excision, but the normal gingival contour must be restored.

Lipoma

The lipoma is a benign connective tissue tumour derived from mature fat cells. It is a common tumour of the subcutaneous tissue and is occasionally found in the mouth. The lipoma is usually a circumscribed, spherical pedunculated mass arising from the oral mucosa. It is found in the submucosa of the cheeks and lips, the tongue and the floor of the mouth (Figure 12.10). The lipoma may be

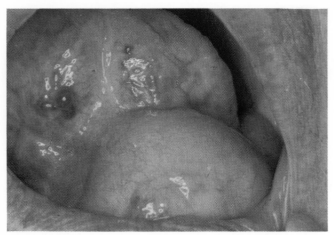

Figure 12.10. *Lipoma presenting in floor of mouth as a large, smooth yellowish swelling.*

multiple and occasionally symmetrically distributed. There is considerable variation in the size of the tumour from several millimetres to several centimetres, when it may then interfere with the patient's normal speech and mastication. When a lipoma occurs in the deep sub-mucosal tissue it appears clinically as a slightly raised pink area, whereas a more superficially situated one is yellow in colour. The deep-seated lipoma may be found on palpation to be a freely movable mass or nodule, or on occasions it may be more diffuse blending with the surrounding tissue. Because of its resilience and spongy texture it is rarely traumatized and ulcerated. Variations do occur, e.g. a fibrolipoma in which there is also a large amount of fibrous tissue or a haemangiolipoma when there is a large col-lection of blood vessels within the tumour. Treatment is by conservative surgical excision; recurrences are rare.

Osteoma

An osteoma is a protruding tumour mass composed of abnormally dense but otherwise normal bone formed by the periosteum; it consists of trabeculae of lamellar bone surrounding fatty or fibrous marrow spaces. These are uncommon tumours almost exclusively involving the skull and facial bones, especially the maxilla or mandible. They are most often seen in patients in the fourth and fifth decades of life. An osteoma is usually asymptomatic, except for the deformity it may cause.

Treatment consists of surgical excision and recurrences are not a problem. The asymptomatic lesion which is not increasing in size need not be removed. Many consider osteomas to be hamartomas (malformations) of bone. The torus palatinus and the torus mandibularis are examples.

In a rare syndrome, Gardner's syndrome, multiple osteomas of the mandible are found in association with osteomas of the calvarium and occasionally of the long bones, with intestinal polyposis and other soft tissue tumours.

Other lesions which may resemble osteomas but which can only be differentiated microscopically are the osteoid osteomas, fibro-osteomas and ossifying fibromas.

Vascular Lesions

Angiomas are among the most common developmental lesions of the oral mucosa. They may be classified broadly as lymphangiomas and haemangiomas, depending upon the type of parent vessel.

Lymphangioma

The lymphangioma is composed of a mass of lymphatic vessels and appears clinically as a pale pink or pink-white lesion, occurring in the tongue or lip. It is usually found at birth or develops early in childhood. The lesion tends to be soft and fluctuant, appearing as a small papillary mass. When deep-seated the appearance will be that of a slightly elevated rubbery mass. The size is variable, and when large may create gross deformity of the oral structures involved, especially in the tongue where it is a cause of macroglossia.

Treatment may be surgical, when excision of the lesion with a wide margin of normal tissue is necessary because there is a marked tendency for it to recur. However, as the lymphangioma is an innocent lesion without malignant potential, surgical intervention may be contraindicated if extensive deformity is likely to result. Sclerosing agents and radiotherapy are used but may not be effective. Occa-sionally, spontaneous regression of the lesion may occur after puberty.

Haemangioma

Haemangiomas are often present at birth or may arise during childhood. The lesion may remain static, or may increase in size as the child grows older, until puberty, when often there is a definite regression. Occasionally, a haemangioma, which has also involved the underlying jaw bone, may be first noticed in an adult patient following tooth extraction which is then followed by haemorrhage.

Clinically, the haemangioma may present in one of sev-eral forms.

1. As a small papillary pedunculated lesion, bright red or purplish in colour, which is often found on the lips, gingiva and tongue (Figure 12.11). It tends to be soft and is easily traumatized with resultant haemorrhage. Clinically, it closely resembles the pyogenic granuloma.

2. A single haemangioma may appear as a raised, sessile, lobulated lesion involving the surface of the mucosa and

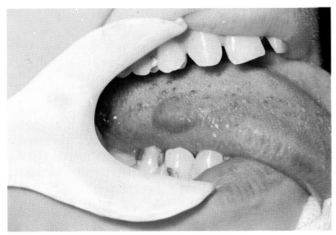

Figure 12.11. *Haemangioma on side of tongue, the bluish coloration indicating that a part is very superficial.*

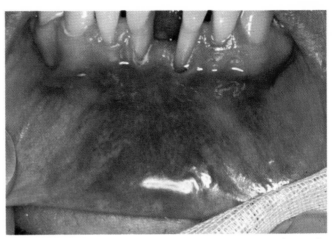

Figure 12.12. *Hereditary haemorrhagic telangiectasia of labial mucosa simulating ecchymoses.*

Figure 12.13. *Hereditary haemorrhagic telangiectasia involving the tongue.*

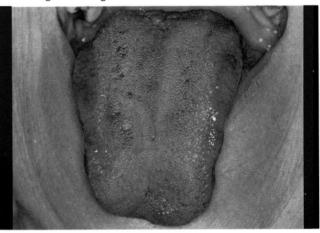

also the deeper submucosal tissues. In some instances the lesion may be firmer and pink if there is a large connective tissue component, as in sclerosing haemangioma.

3. Large, irregular, slightly raised purplish lesions are usually found on the buccal mucosa, where their distribution tends to be extensive. These lesions present a multicentric pattern, numerous distinct lesions joining to cover a large area. Depending on the amount of blood present in vascular spaces the lesion tends to appear raised or flat and blanches on pressure.

Treatment of haemangiomas depends on several factors such as the age of the patient, the size of the lesion and clinical character. It may include surgery, radiotherapy, or sclerosing agents.

Syndromes with Vascular Oral Lesions

Osler–Rendu–Parkes–Weber Syndrome

Hereditary haemorrhagic telangiectasia or angiomatosis is a familial disorder characterized by angiomas appearing at puberty or later in life. Sites affected are usually the lips, oral mucosa (Figure 12.12), tongue (Figure 12.13), facial skin, conjunctiva, nasal and pharyngeal mucosa. The lesions are small appearing as minute deep-red papules, and are microscopically haemangiomas of the capillaries with occasional larger cavernous spaces. Haemorrhage is a common problem from any area involved, e.g. oral cavity, gastrointestinal tract, respiratory tract.

Sturge–Weber Syndrome

This is a neurocutaneous syndrome with occasional lesions of the oral mucosa (Figure 12.14). There is

Figure 12.14. *Phenytoin hyperplasia superimposed on a case of Sturge–Weber syndrome. The gingiva here is a much deeper plum colour in contrast to the appearance of phenytoin hyperplasia alone.*

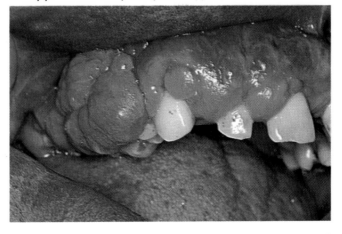

angiomatosis of the skin and of the mucosa as well as of the leptomeninges. Cutaneous lesions are usually unilateral and appear on the face as a large deep-red haemangioma which may extend deeply into the subcutaneous tissue. The meningeal lesions often contain calcified laminated concretions readily seen on skull radiographs. Epilepsy, mental retardation, and hemiplegia may occur in certain cases.

Neurofibroma

The neurofibroma is a tumour that arises from all the sheath elements of a peripheral nerve, and may be solitary or multiple as part of the von Recklinghausen—neurofibromatosis syndrome.

The single lesion is a developmental malformation and may occur in any part of the mouth, especially in the tongue, buccal mucosa, floor of the mouth (Figure 12.15)

Figure 12.15. *Neurofibroma in floor of mouth closely related to opening of submandibular and sublingual salivary glands.*

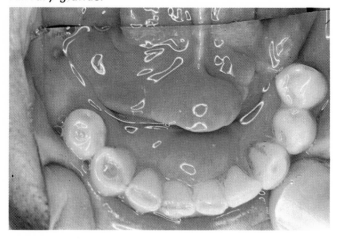

and the palate. It is frequently seen in children. Clinically, it may appear as a pedunculated firm growth but more usually it is found as a firm nodule, partly submerged and slightly movable. Often on palpation it may be found not to be well circumscribed but to merge with the surrounding tissue.

Treatment consists of surgical excision, but there is always the problem of severing a nerve. In a large oral neurofibroma in childhood it is usual to wait until puberty before carrying out surgery, but then the diagnosis should be confirmed by biopsy at an early stage. Occasionally some of these lesions may undergo regression, while others may undergo cystic degeneration.

Von Recklinghausen's Neurofibromatosis

Von Recklinghausen's neurofibromatosis consists of multiple neurofibromas of the skin and other tissues, plus discrete areas of melanin pigmentation of the skin (café au lait spots). The oral mucosa is invariably involved with the nerve lesions, particularly the tongue, gingiva, and labial mucosa, but there is no oral pigmentation. Malignant alteration of skin and deeper tumours is reasonably frequent, and once this has occurred the prognosis is relatively poor because of early metastases.

Conclusion

It will be seen from this account that many of these benign lesions of the mouth have similar features clinically, and the definitive diagnosis is frequently impossible without a biopsy. It may also be said that the initial stages of malignant lesions in this site may present with similar features and be relatively symptomless. This emphasizes the importance of early referral of patients for immediate biopsy and appropriate treatment, and frequently saves the patient a great deal of trouble in the long term.

13. Malignant Neoplasms

C. C. Rachanis

Oral cancer is a disease with a very poor prognosis. About 40 per cent of patients are dead within a year of commencing treatment (Binnie et al. 1972). Of all cancer registrations in England and Wales about two per cent relate to oral malignant neoplasms and they account for one in every 100 cancer deaths. More than half of all patients with intra-oral cancer present themselves for treatment at a late stage of the disease, and consequently have a poor prognosis. This is most unfortunate when one considers that the mouth is easily accessible for inspection, biopsy and treatment whether by radiotherapy or surgery. In some countries, for example in India and South-East Asia, the incidence is much higher, being about 25 to 47 per cent of all cancers.

Carcinoma

Squamous cell (epidermoid) carcinoma of the oral mucosa is the most commonly occurring malignant neoplasm in the oral cavity, accounting for about 95 per cent of all malignant growths in the mouth. Other forms of carcinoma, including that of the salivary glands, plus the primary malignant mesenchymal tumours and secondary deposits make up the remaining five per cent. Rarely does carcinoma occur in the jaws as a primary tumour. The vast majority of carcinomas affecting the jaws are either tumours of adjacent structures which have involved the bone by direct extension, or they are secondary deposits from growths at some distant site, e.g. breast, lung, kidney, etc.

Incidence

The peak incidence in the UK and the USA is from 55 to 75 years of age, whereas in India it is from 40 to 45 years of age; cases below 30 years of age have been reported in a few instances. With regard to the sex incidence there is a definite male preponderance varying in degree for tumours occurring at the different sites, e.g. ratio of 14:1

for lip lesions and 4:1 for lesions in the floor of the mouth. In Scandinavian countries, however, a relatively higher proportion of females suffer from carcinoma of the tongue and pharynx. This may be related to the prevalence of the Paterson–Kelly syndrome in those countries.

Sites of Occurrence

Squamous cell carcinoma can occur anywhere in the mouth, but certain sites appear to be more frequently involved than others. Information about sites of origin generally refers to the five major structures of the mouth, namely, the tongue, the mucosa of the cheek, the floor of the mouth, the hard and soft palates and the gingiva. Studies over the years have shown that there is a rough guide for the location of oral carcinoma. The following list outlines the most commonly affected sites.

1. One-quarter of cancerous lesions occur in each of the two alveolar–lingual sulcus areas, i.e. the posterior part of the floor of the mouth between the tongue and the alveolar ridge.

2. One-quarter of cases occur in the more anterior portion of the floor of the mouth.

3. The remaining one-quarter is scattered throughout all other areas of the mouth.

Thus there are two main areas where about 70 per cent of all cases are located. Carcinomas in various sites will differ in their clinical appearance, rate of growth, metastasis and prognosis. However, there are different racial patterns.

Aetiology

As with other forms of cancer the aetiology of squamous cell carcinoma is still unknown, but in recent years, through experimental work and the application of epidemiological techniques using incidence patterns, some understanding has been obtained of the complex

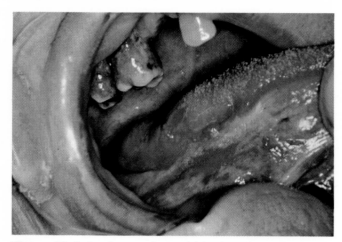

Figure 13.1. *Lesion on lateral border of tongue and floor of mouth which was painless and on clinical examination was ulcerated and indurated. Clinical appearance was suggestive of cancer; biopsy showed it to be a squamous cell carcinoma.*

Figure 13.2. *Biopsy of this lesion confirmed the clinical impression of carcinoma. It was found to be a verrucous carcinoma.*

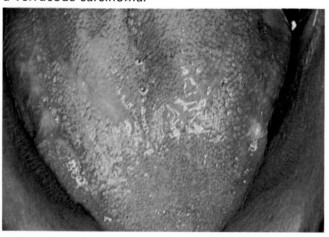

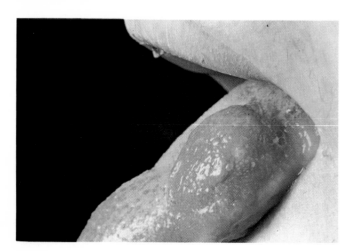

factors involved in the development of malignant tumours in general, and in the oral cavity in particular. Although the fundamental cause remains unknown, some stimulating or predisposing factors can be recognized. The most commonly suspected of these factors in the development of oral cancer appear to be:

1. Tobacco smoking and tobacco chewing.

2. Chronic alcohol consumption.

3. Nutritional deficiencies, e.g. Paterson–Kelly syndrome, malnutrition.

4. Sunlight, particularly in relation to lip cancer.

5. Syphilis.

6. Ionizing radiation, as a long-term complication of radiotherapy.

7. Miscellaneous factors such as trauma, poor oral hygiene, sepsis, chronic irritation from jagged teeth and dentures—all of these factors are not thought to be significant, including submucous fibrosis and betel-nut chewing. An increased incidence has also been found to occur in the lower socioeconomic groups.

It is difficult to give a typical description of oral carcinoma because the clinical appearance is far from uniform. The clinician must become acquainted with the numerous varied clinical features exhibited by this malignant lesion, and the information obtained from epidemiological studies characterizing the tumours, e.g. location, age, sex, race, size, premalignant conditions, occupation, habits, etc., and also develop a high index of suspicion, particularly of surface changes of the oral mucosa. This is made all the more difficult because there are very many benign lesions which also manifest changes of the surface mucosa, and thus early cancer is often misdiagnosed for one of these lesions and not recognized for what it is.

Clinical Types

On examination, carcinoma may appear in the early stages to have developed into one of the following clinical types:

1. Ulcerative type—this is the most frequent type and on occasions has been erroneously diagnosed as acute ulcerative gingivitis (Vincent's infection), or as traumatic ulceration caused by the flange of an ill-fitting denture (Figure 13.1). Typically the ulcer is indurated and sometimes has firm everted or rolled edges.

2. Papillary or verrucous type (Figure 13.2). The growth is

Figure 13.3. *(Left) Elevated nodular lesion not associated with any recognizable causative agent; it was painless and indurated. Biopsy confirmed an infiltrating squamous cell carcinoma.*

soft, wartlike and may be extensive, particularly on the cheek.

3. Nodular type (Figure 13.3). The growth starts as a firm nodule apparently under the mucosa, which is slowly growing and may eventually ulcerate.

4. Deeply infiltrating or scirrhous type, infiltrating the deeper structures without much surface change.

5. As a white raised plaque, which may proliferate and become fissured. Later there may be ulceration of the expanding lesion (Figure 13.4).

Apart from the patient's awareness of a swelling or ulcer or the disturbance in the fit of a denture, symptoms of oral cancer are few until a late stage in the disease. Pain is not a feature of these growths unless major nerve bundles are involved.

Not infrequently the patient may complain of an enlarged cervical lymph node which is found to be painless and firm. This too often arises late in the progress of the tumour unless it is poorly differentiated. The most common signs of intra-oral carcinoma are induration, ulceration, fungation (Figure 13.5), fixation and mobility of teeth when alveolar bone is destroyed.

Metastatic Spread

Metastatic spread is usually via the lymphatic vessels to the regional lymph nodes. The frequency of metastases depends on the site, size and differentiation of the primary tumour. The prognosis is related to the size of the primary lesion and to the degree of lymph node involvement. The site offering the best prognosis is the lip, mainly because a carcinoma here is noticed and diagnosed at an earlier stage than in other sites. In contrast, carcinoma of the posterior third of the tongue is usually detected at a much later stage, is therefore much larger when noticed, less well differentiated, and has a greater tendency to lymph node spread, often bilaterally, and is complicated by the relatively greater problems of surgical access.

According to Storer (1972) late diagnosis may be made because 75 per cent of cases occur in people over 60 years of age, and a very high proportion of these are edentulous. These elderly edentulous patients, who do not usually attend for regular oral examinations, are satisfied provided the dentures are not causing discomfort, and are often conditioned to expect minor irritations associated with them. Often in the past, ulceration caused by the denture has healed without help from the dentist. In consequence, a new and now neoplastic lesion may be neglected by the patient. There is also a large number of elderly and chronically sick patients in geriatric units, psychiatric hospitals, voluntary homes or other institutions where they are unlikely to see a dentist unless referred by a physician.

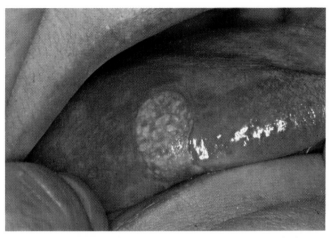

Figure 13.4. *Well-circumscribed ulcerated nodular type of carcinoma of lateral border of tongue. Note mucosal surface changes distal to the lesion indicative of extension of the lesion.*

Figure 13.5. *Fungating carcinoma involving the posterior parts of upper and lower alveolar ridges, part of soft palate and anterior faucial pillar.*

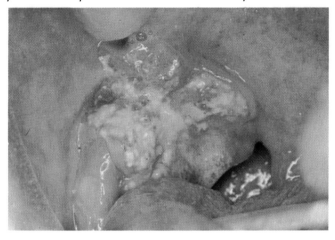

Treatment

Treatment of oral carcinoma at present involves radiation, surgery, or a combination of both depending upon the histology of the biopsy, the size and site of the neoplasm, its radiosensitivity, degree of metastases and the age and physical condition of the patient. The treatment of choice is radiotherapy when it produces better results than surgery, when surgery is contraindicated, when functional results may be better with irradiation even though the survival rate may be similar and when irradiation produces satisfactory palliation. Ionizing radiation can be

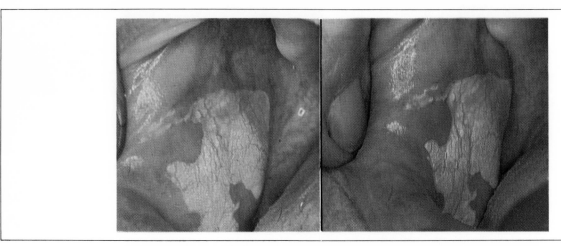

Figure 13.6. *Homogeneous leukoplakia involving the cheek mucosa bilaterally. Very similar in appearance to one of the types of lichen planus. Diagnosis confirmed by biopsy.*

administered either externally by deep x-ray machine or mega voltage units, or internally by radium or other implants.

In a well-differentiated and reasonably small carcinoma local excision with an adequate margin of healthy tissue suffices, and the patient should be kept under close observation. In a larger but well-differentiated carcinoma the surgical approach is more radical and when palpable lymph nodes are found, block dissection of the neck is indicated. With clinical or radiographic evidence of invasion into osseous tissue resection of bone is necessary. Inoperability may be determined by the following:

1. Histology showing the tumour to be anaplastic.

2. Extensive neck lymph node involvement and/or the presence of distant metastases.

3. Poor general condition of the patient.

Chemotherapy so far has proved of little effect in the control of oral malignant disease.

Leukoplakia

Leukoplakia (= 'white plaque') may be defined as any white patch or plaque, not less than 5 mm in diameter, which cannot be removed by rubbing and which cannot be classified as any other diagnosable disease (Figure 13.6). This is a clinical definition and carries no histological connotation. Unfortunately, the term carries implications of malignant potential, and yet a number of benign lesions are characterized by the formation of white patches and are only very rarely associated with the subsequent appearance of malignancy.

Incidence

It occurs more frequently in males than females, and the aetiological factors are probably similar to those suggested for carcinoma of the oral mucosa. The lesions show considerable variation in size, location, clinical appearance, and behaviour. Certain sites of predilection have been noted, e.g. cheek mucosa, angles of the mouth, alveolar mucosa, tongue (Figure 13.7), lip, hard and soft palates and floor of mouth, in descending order of frequency. On examination the white patches may vary from a non-palpable, faintly translucent whitish area to thick, fissured, papillary indurated lesions. There is a definite relationship of leukoplakia to carcinoma with malignancy following leukoplakia in a proportion of cases (Figure 13.8). There is difficulty in deciding which lesions are likely to undergo malignant transformation, but it has been noted that the speckled or nodular form is more likely to progress in this direction. Occasionally frank carcinoma may present with the appearance of leukoplakia, underlining the fact that the definition is a clinical one lacking histological precision. This emphasizes the desirability of biopsying all white patches to exclude malignancy.

Aetiology

Smoking, especially a pipe and cigars, is often associated with the appearance of a slight to moderate diffuse white or grey appearance of the entire palate. The posterior half is usually covered with white umbilicated papules having red centres, which correspond with the openings of the mucous gland ducts. This condition is known under a

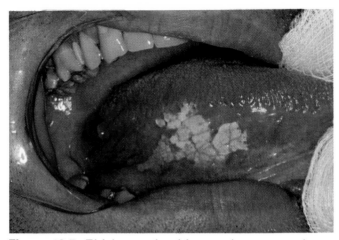

Figure 13.7. *Thick, rough white patch on ventral surface of tongue which could not be rubbed off. Biopsy confirmed diagnosis of leukoplakia.*

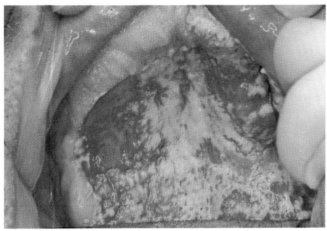

Figure 13.8. *Leukoplakia of palate which has undergone malignant transformation to squamous cell carcinoma. May originally have started as stomatitis nicotina.*

variety of terms such as smoker's keratosis, stomatitis nicotina and strawberry palate (Figure 13.9). It is most severe in heavy smokers and improves when smoking is discontinued. In denture wearers those portions of the palate protected by a denture do not develop these white patches.

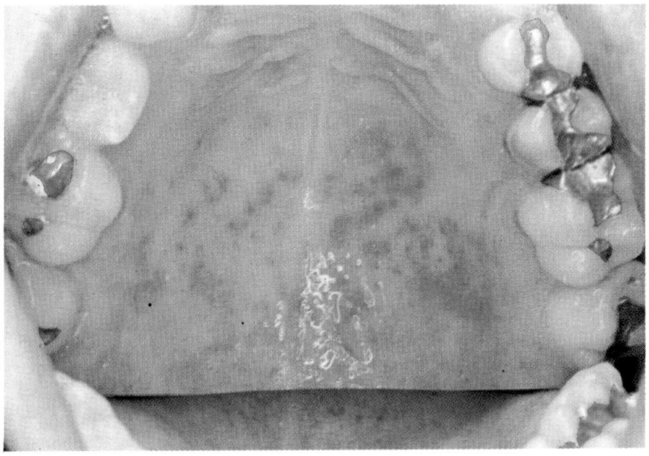

Ameloblastoma (Adamantinoma)

The ameloblastoma, a rare tumour, arises from the epithelial component of the odontogenic tissues (tooth-forming tissues). It behaves as a locally malignant tumour. 'Adamantinoma' is inappropriate because the tumour does not contain formed enamel, as the odontogenic epithelium fails to undergo differentiation to the point of enamel formation. Indeed, it is often soft and cystic in nature.

Figure 13.9. *Diffuse white patch of palate with umbilicated papules containing red centres, the openings of the mucous glands, in a heavy smoker.*

Incidence

It accounts for approximately one per cent of all oral tumours, with a slight but insignificant male preponderance of cases. Most ameloblastomas are found in patients between 20 and 50 years of age, with a peak incidence of detection occurring about 35 years of age. Because it is very slow growing the tumour will often have been present for some appreciable time before diagnosis. About 80 per cent originate in the mandible, with nearly three-quarters of these occurring at the angle of the mandible in the molar region and/or the ramus. The maxilla is less commonly affected, with lesions in the molar regions, the antrum and the floor of the nose. According to various studies this tumour is thought to occur more frequently in Africans than in Caucasians.

Symptoms and Signs

The ameloblastoma begins insidiously as a central lesion within bone existing for several years before symptoms develop. It does not often produce signs or symptoms of nerve involvement and is seldom painful unless secondarily infected. At this early stage of development the tumour is usually found during routine radiographic examination of the jaws. It is slowly destructive tending

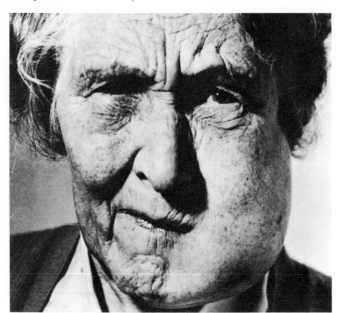

Figure 13.10. *Gross facial deformity caused by presence of ameloblastoma at left angle of the mandible.*

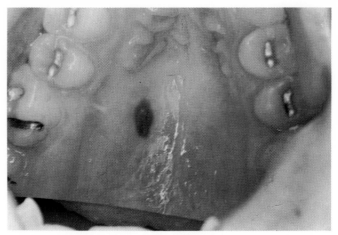

Figure 13.11. *Malignant melanoma of hard palate showing deepening of coloration, but no ulceration.*

later to expand the bone rather than perforate through it to the oral tissues, which is a late feature when it occurs. Examination may reveal facial deformity (Figure 13.10). The swelling at first is bony hard and covered by normal mucous membrane or skin. In time the alveolus or even the entire jaw is expanded and the cortical bone, usually the buccal plate, becomes thinned so that local pressure may elicit eggshell crackling or even fluctuation. Displacement, loosening or exfoliation of teeth in the region of the tumour may also be observed. If one of these teeth is extracted the tumour will tend to extend into the socket, become infected and cause pain. Occasionally patients are found with an ameloblastoma they have had for many years without seeking treatment, and, although the expansion has been gross and disfiguring, there is seldom breakdown of the oral mucosa. The fungating, ulcerative type of growth which is characteristic of oral carcinoma does not occur.

Radiologically the lesion causes polycystic or monocystic destruction of bone, the former showing well-defined radiolucent areas presenting a honeycomb or soap-bubble appearance and signs of jaw expansion. However, these appearances are not restricted to the ameloblastoma for they may be found in giant cell lesions and some non-neoplastic cysts of the jaws.

Prognosis

The prognosis for patients with this form of neoplastic disease is favourable, even in late cases, but there may be varying degrees of disfigurement. It is essentially a locally destructive lesion and it seldom causes death unless vital structures are involved by local invasion.

Treatment

The ameloblastoma is resistant to radiotherapy. Surgical resection of the tumour including a wide margin of normal bone on all sides, or even hemimandibulectomy, are the treatments of choice because recurrences after adequate surgery are unusual. Regardless of the form of treatment employed, it is essential that long-term follow-up of the patient be maintained for a recurrent lesion may not become obvious until many years after initial treatment.

Malignant Melanoma

The malignant melanoma is an uncommon neoplasm of the oral mucosa. It occurs twice as frequently in males as in females, with a peak incidence between 55 and 65 years of age, and a definite predilection for the maxillary alveolar ridge and palate (Figure 13.11). The tumour appears as a dark brown or bluish-black area which may be slightly elevated, or it may be a larger mass with a nodular or papillary surface, but painless. On rare occasions the lesion may be devoid of pigment. The lesion is frequently asymptomatic and unnoticed until metastatic regional lymph nodes are detected. Often the patient's attention is only drawn to its presence when ulceration and bleeding occur. The appearance of melanin pigmentation in the mouth (not of racial or developmental origin), its increase in size and deepening coloration should be viewed suspiciously, for it has been noted that in about 30 per cent of all cases this type of behaviour has preceded the development of the

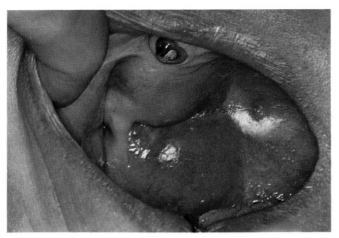

Figure 13.12. *Lymphosarcoma of the soft palate and anterior faucial pillar, with the typical soft, red, fleshy appearance.*

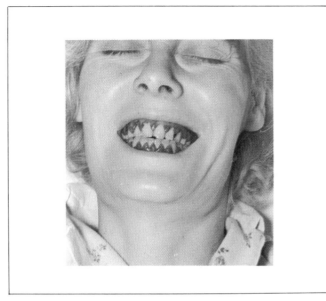

Figure 13.13. *Swollen, deeply red gingiva in a case of acute monocytic leukaemia.*

neoplasm. Growth is rapid, with invasion and extensive destruction of bone, accompanied by loosening of teeth and metastases to the regional lymph nodes and distant sites.

Sarcoma

A sarcoma is a malignant tumour arising from any mesenchymal tissue. The prefixes fibro-, osteo-, lipo-, etc., indicate the specific tissue of origin (Figure 13.12). A sarcoma is more likely to appear in children and young adults, whereas carcinoma is a tumour appearing in later life, particularly in the mouth. Sarcomas vary greatly in malignant behaviour depending on the tissue from which they arise. They are rare tumours of the mouth, and have a very poor prognosis. Metastases take place via the bloodstream and are found at distant sites, e.g. large vital organs especially in the lungs. Occasionally a sarcoma is found in the mouth having metastasized from a primary lesion elsewhere. The development of sarcoma in an area of Paget's disease is a well-known complication, but jaw tumours are rare.

Leukaemia

Oral manifestations of leukaemia are more dramatic and occur more frequently in the acute forms, in about 55 per cent of cases of acute leukaemia and in approximately 15 per cent of cases of the chronic disease. A patient may present for the treatment of oral lesions which may appear to be local in nature.

Symptoms and Signs

The primary clinical manifestations of acute leukaemia most commonly involve the gingiva and include gingivitis, gingival enlargement, haemorrhage and ulceration. The gingival enlargement which is a constant feature is usually generalized and of varying severity. In severe cases it may cover the greater part of the crowns of the teeth. The gingiva will be found to be swollen, soft and spongy, oedematous, deep red to cyanotic in colour, and will tend to bleed very easily (Figure 13.13). A great deal of the swelling is caused by the intensive leukaemic cell infiltration. This is especially noticeable in areas where there is mild chronic irritation. Gingival haemorrhage is caused by ulceration of the crevicular epithelium of the sulcus. Ulceration and necrosis of the underlying tissues are the result of depression of the normal inflammatory response of the gingival tissues to the ever-present mild infection, because the immature white cells are ineffective in combating this. White cell thrombosis in the gingival vessels also contributes. Therefore, in many instances a patient may present initially with what appears to be a severe acute ulcerative gingivitis (Vincent's infection, AUG, trench mouth), and/or with ulceration of other parts of the oral mucous membrane.

With pathological changes taking place in the periodontium, through thrombosis of periodontal vessels and necrosis of alveolar bone, rapid loosening of teeth occurs, occasionally accompanied by pain. Extraction of such teeth will result in continuous and often profuse post-extraction haemorrhage, which may also occur as a primary manifestation. Other manifestations are the appearance of petechiae and ecchymoses, especially in those areas of the oral mucosa that are easily traumatized.

In the chronic forms of leukaemia the manifestations are less dramatic with the gingival reaction again predominating but with much less discomfort. All the various oral manifestations discussed for the acute form of leukaemia may be noted.

Treatment

Local therapy is very important and may afford considerable relief to a patient with troublesome oral lesions. Simple periodontal procedures such as removal of soft deposits from the teeth will help alleviate much of the local inflammatory response which is mainly an exaggeration of a pre-existing gingivitis. Frequent irrigations or mouthwashes with warm saline or weak hydrogen peroxide solutions are soothing and help remove exudate, necrotic tissue and recently acquired food particles from the interdental areas. Occasionally antibiotic (including a fungicide) mouthwashes may have to be prescribed to treat coexistent oral infections especially oral candidiasis, e.g. Mysteclin (tetracycline and nystatin).

References

Binnie, W. H., Cawson, R. A., Hill, G. B. and Soper, A., *Oral Cancer in England and Wales*, HMSO, 1972.
Storer, R., *Lancet*, 1972, **i**, 430.

Section 5
Looking at the Throat

14. The Oropharynx, Nasopharynx, Laryngopharynx and Larynx

R. F. McNab Jones

Examination of the oropharynx, the nasopharynx, the laryngopharynx and larynx presents different problems — each area will therefore be considered separately.

The Oropharynx

The oropharynx includes the pillars of the fauces, the tonsils in front, the soft palate and uvula above, the pharynx and dorsum of the tongue down to the upper edge of the epiglottis below, and the area of posterior pharyngeal wall seen when the soft palate is elevated in phonation. The whole area is covered in stratified squamous epithelium of a uniform pink colour. Submucosal vessels are particularly well seen on the dorsum of the tongue and posterior pharyngeal wall. Before examination of these areas, the patient should be asked to remove any dentures.

Examination

All are familiar with the traditional spatula and light examination and the exhortation to say 'aah'. Familiarity may breed a degree of slackness in this exercise and we should recall its exact purpose. On asking a patient to open his mouth wide, a variable amount of the oropharynx is visible. Usually the upper third of the fauces and tonsil and a small area of the posterior pharyngeal wall can be glimpsed above the dorsum of the tongue. Even at this stage of the examination difficulties may arise. Trismus can prevent any proper view of the area, while in a few hypersensitive patients even this simple request causes gagging (Figure 14.1). Asking the patient to protrude the tongue rarely improves the view of the oropharynx, but can give useful information about the condition of the tongue and its mobility (Figure 14.2). These two steps in the examination should precede the insertion of a spatula.

The spatula is used to depress the tongue and ideally should be angled so that the hand holding it does not obstruct one's view. Insert it slowly and gently, not further than half way along the dorsum of the tongue in the first instance, and be sure the patient is not protruding the tongue as many tend to do at this point. Depress it slowly, relaxing the pressure if gagging results, until the lower

Figure 14.1. *Palatal swelling, showing a restricted view of a typical quinsy.*

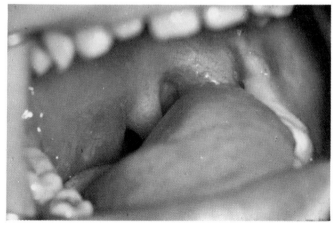

Figure 14.2. *Reticulosis at the base of the tongue.*

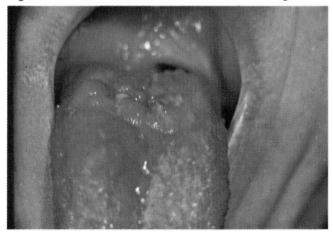

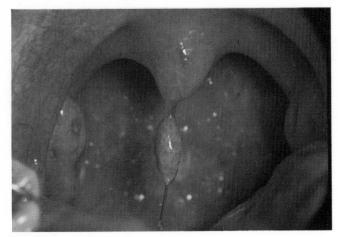

Figure 14.3. *Papilloma of the uvula.*

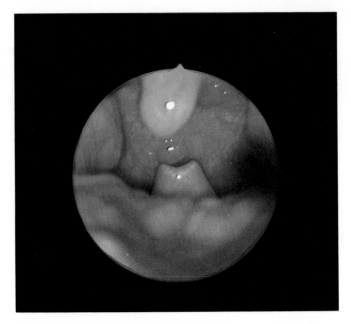

Figure 14.4. *View of the uvula, tongue and epiglottis in a patient 10 years of age.*

Figure 14.5. *Antrochoanal polypi seen in the oropharynx. Some conditions of the nasopharynx can be seen on ordinary examination of the mouth.*

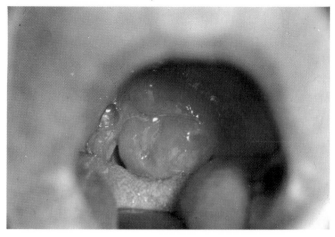

limits of the tonsillar fossa are visible. One should now have a good view of the vallate papillae and dorsum of the tongue, and a wide area of the posterior pharyngeal wall; perhaps one can just see the tip of the epiglottis. When the patient says 'aah', two main changes occur. The posterior pillars of the fauces move towards the mid-line, opening up the tonsillar fossi for better inspection and 'squeezing' any lymphoid tissue on the lateral pharyngeal walls into a more prominent and obvious position. The soft palate is raised and more of the posterior pharyngeal wall becomes visible (Figure 14.3).

In this phase of the examination one should be looking at:

1. The condition of the dorsum of the tongue.

2. The anterior and posterior faucial pillars, their appearance and movement.

3. The tonsils, especially as seen when the patient phonates, their size, state of the crypts, any swellings, ulceration, pus or foreign bodies.

4. The state of the tip of the epiglottis if visible. This is particularly well seen in children (Figure 14.4).

5. The posterior pharyngeal wall.

6. The appearance of the soft palate and uvula and its movements. Does it close the oropharynx adequately from the nasopharynx on phonation? Are there any abnormalities in its movements?

Further means of examination can be used if necessary. Any ulcer or swelling should be palpated and its consistency and mobility noted. If a head light or mirror are used for illumination, two hands are free for instruments. While depressing the tongue with one hand, use another angled tongue depressor to retract the anterior pillar of the fauces and gently squeeze the tonsil. This may reveal

previously unseen pathology and the presence of pus in the tonsil crypts. Two hands are also necessary for the removal of foreign bodies in the area.

Particular difficulties in the examination can be met with in infants and children and in adults with hypersensitive throats. Infants must be wrapped tightly in a blanket and examined lying down while an assistant holds the infant's head steady. Gentle insertion of the spatula will cause gagging and this allows a reasonably extensive though brief view of the area. The same ruse can be used to view recalcitrant children. In hypersensitive adults, the use of a local anaesthetic spray may be helpful.

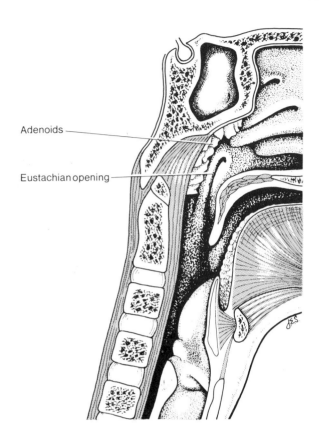

Adenoids

Eustachian opening

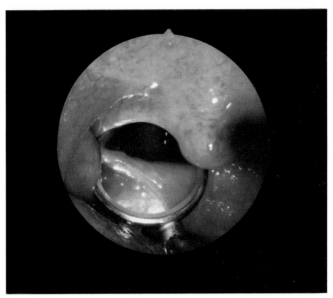

Figure 14.7. *Approach to the postnasal space.*

Figure 14.6. *(a) (Above) Section through the nasopharynx. (b) (Below) Examination of the postnasal space. (Inset: view in mirror.)*

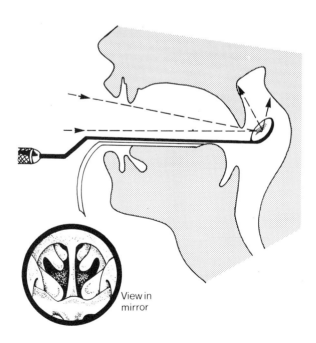

View in mirror

As most of this area can be seen and palpated, radiography or other methods of examination are rarely necessary.

The Nasopharynx (Postnasal Space)

Examination

Usually this area (Figure 14.5) is examined with the aid of a small angled mirror held in the oropharynx and tilted in various directions to provide views of the whole area (Figure 14.6, a and b). The mirror should be warmed slightly before use to stop misting and must be inserted very carefully so as to avoid touching adjacent parts (Figure 14.7). Roughly 50 per cent of patients will gag during this examination and prevent an adequate view of the area being obtained. Some of these can be examined more successfully after spraying the throat with a local anaesthetic.

Considerable experience is required to interpret the findings. Under good conditions the examiner can see the posterior choanae with the white posterior edge of the septum a prominent landmark, and the posterior ends of the turbinates seen in each choana (Figure 14.8). The posterior end of the inferior turbinates is often enlarged and sometimes forms a considerable 'mulberry' swelling which obstructs the nasal airway. The anterior arch of the atlas forms a variable-sized bulge on the posterior pharyngeal wall and the openings of the eustachian tubes are visible low down on each lateral wall.

A useful additional investigation is a lateral soft tissue x-ray of the area when any encroachment on the airway is clearly visible (Figure 14.9).

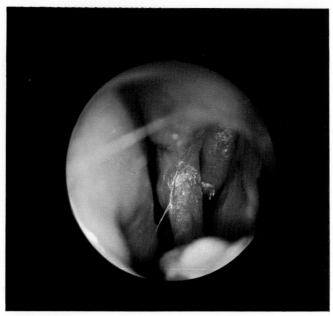

Figure 14.8. *Mirror view of postnasal space.*

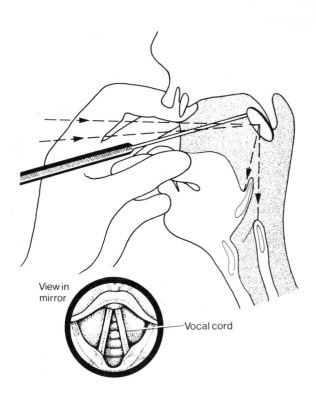

Figure 14.10. *Indirect laryngoscopy.*

Figure 14.9. *X-ray of postnasal space showing enlargement of adenoids.*

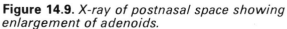
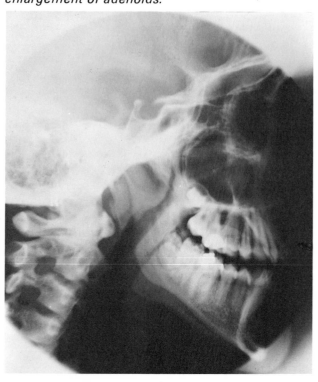

When necessary the area may also be examined under an anaesthetic. The patient is usually laid on his back and a Boyle–Davis type gag inserted. After elevating the soft palate with rubber catheters drawn tight through the nose and mouth, a medium-sized angled mirror is placed in the oropharynx. Instrumental or digital palpation may also help at this stage.

The Pharynx and Larynx

Examination

Outpatient examination is done by means of a large angled mirror as shown in Figure 14.10. The area is first viewed during gentle respiration and then with the patient saying 'eee'. Phonation raises the soft palate and the larynx, which also tilts forwards. This makes it possible to see into the anterior half of the glottis. In the average patient an adequate view of the following parts is obtained and each should be consciously checked over:

1. Dorsum of tongue, vallecula and anterior surface of epiglottis.

2. Tip of epiglottis and any ariglottic folds.

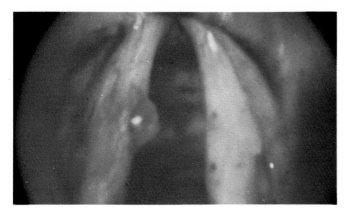

Figure 14.11. *Inflamed polyp of the vocal cord.*

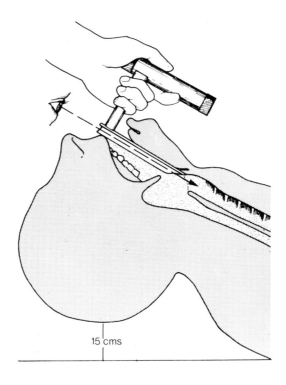

15 cms

Figure 14.12. *Direct laryngoscopy.*

3. The upper half of each pyriform fossa. A deeper view into the fossae is obtained when the patient phonates.

4. The arytenoid cartilages and a small amount of the postcricoid region. The best view of this area is also obtained on phonation.

5. The interior of the larynx showing vestibular folds; a little of the vestibule; the upper surface of the vocal cords. Special attention must be paid to the appearance and movements of the vocal cords (Figure 14.11). On deep inspiration, the cords abduct and a variable amount of the subglottic area and upper trachea are visible through the open glottis.

In patients with a sensitive pharynx, local anaesthesia may be required. It should be possible to obtain an adequate view of the area in about 80 per cent of patients.

Additional methods of examination include plain x-rays where the lateral view is most helpful. Tomography is more informative and can be performed in the AP or lateral positions.

In patients in whom a proper view cannot be obtained by the above methods or when palpation or biopsy of the area is required, direct laryngoscopy (Figure 14.12) under a general anaesthetic is necessary.

Mirror examination of the pharynx and larynx is not easy. For those with little experience, attempts to 'look at' these areas are unrewarding and may be misleading.

Index